T0214664

'It has been a privilege to review this textbook as it is prepared for publishing, and to encourage all who encounter it to read it not as a text to quote but as a challenge to the status quo of your life. Johanna pushes us to think, to consider ways of knowing, to be brave, to challenge systems that are not or may not be safe (or working well enough for those they serve). Johanna encourages us to consider the beauty of the whole that is in front of us and to respond to that one, not a carbon copy or a text book description of a person. Read with your mind ready to be challenged, and then respond by thinking deeply about the concepts and pictures that she offers. You will be reminded of the times that you have not felt safe, and this excellent book will help you to recognise how others might have less of this experience in the future in our health care systems. My hope is that this expands into Life as you consider alternate ways of being with many others in your daily round.'

Carolyn Russell MBBS FRACGP, Dip RACOG Mast Social Science (Counselling); GP psychotherapist; Medical Educator and Supervisor for GPTQ, RACGP, and MPS/Cognitive Institute

'The time for restoring the generalist craft of healing-centered care has arrived, and Johanna Lynch's *A Whole Person Approach to Well-Being: Building a Sense of Safety* will serve as a foundational text for generalism's renewal. A good word, sewn well, becomes a fruitful seed. A community of good words, carefully chosen, transform a landscape into an ecology of healing. Johanna Lynch offers us a basket of such words with an engaging style that will motivate you to join in seeding the field of generalism and begin nourishing and growing our collective well-being. *A Whole Person Approach to Well-Being* is a book about words, generative words, and a book about growth, growth into a "sense of safety," written for generalist healers and teachers who use words to help others and themelves grow sense and safety. We learn to move from "nouns of distress" to "verbs of well-being," and how to simultaneously use words that widen, connect, and integrate. Intellectually stunning, carefully crafted, grounded in decades of deep clinical experience, filled with heart-opening stories and indigenous wisdom, imaginative, and exceptionally well-written, Johanna Lynch's *A Whole Person Approach to Well-Being* also welcomes its readers to a festival celebrating and re-imagining the transdisciplinary generalist craft of healing-centered care. Pursuing a pathway for transforming whole person and whole community care, Johanna Lynch offers us the metaphorically rich and physiologically powerful "sense of safety" as a healing goal. Readers will learn the importance of eye juggling awareness of self, other, and context in search of that sense of safety that protects integrity, connection, and coherence. As a family physician and teacher of future generalist healers, and transdisciplinary, mixed methods primary care researcher for over thirty-five years, I am, after reading this book, looking wider and making changes to my craft. Come, engage the words in this book, and discover the magic that happens when a wide scope, relational process, healing purpose, and integrative wisdom combine in Johanna Lynch's cauldron and a sense of safety emerges.'

William L. Miller, MD, MA, Chair Emeritus of Family Medicine Lehigh Valley Health Network; Professor of Family Medicine University of South Florida Morsani College of Medicine

'Johanna Lynch's wonderful book brings valuable new insights into why generalist care is so important: as a means of generating and maintaining a sense of safety for our many patients who consult with us in distress. Working towards that sense of safety gives generalists a profound moral purpose, a convincing rationale for why we do what we do. Lynch offers us and our patients, together, a coherent understanding of the integration of different elements of the person, not just our bodily experiences, but also our environment, our relationships and our inner sense of meaning. With sensitive case studies drawn from the author's own life story, and from her experiences as a family doctor with special expertise in trauma care, she encourages us to reflect on key questions and pointers for action: about finding places and people to help us feel safe; about calming our bodies; and about how we can hold on to hope.'

Christopher Dowrick BA MSc MD FRCGP, Professor of Primary Medical Care, University of Liverpool, UK; Chair of Working Party for Mental Health, World Organisation of Family Doctors (WONCA)

'Johanna Lynch's book is a precious resource for ambitious primary care clinicians who strive not only to cure and fix in the narrow sense, but to understand, and heal. Sense of safety represents a powerful "threshold concept"; once you have grasped its meaning and scope, there is no way back to not knowing. The argument is innovative, meticulous, and in full accord with contemporary evidence and theory, ranging from cellular biology to existential philosophy. Read this book!'

Linn Getz, MD, PhD, Professor in Behavioral Sciences in Medicine and Leader of the General Practice Research Unit, Norwegian University of Science and Technology

A Whole Person Approach to Wellbeing

This book builds on the person-centred medicine movement to promote a shift in the philosophy of care of distress. It discusses the vital importance of whole person health, healing and growth. Developing a new transdisciplinary concept of *sense of safety*, this book argues that the whole person needs to be understood within their context and relationships and explores the appraisal and coping systems that are part of health.

Using clinical vignettes to illustrate her argument, Lynch draws on an understanding of attachment and trauma-informed approaches to life story and counsels against an over-reliance on symptom-based fragmentation of body and mind.

Integrating literature from social determinants of health, psychology, psychotherapy, education and the social sciences with new research from the fields of immunology, endocrinology and neurology, this broad-ranging book is relevant to all those with an interest in person-centred healthcare, including academics and practitioners from medicine, nursing, mental health and public health.

Johanna Lynch is a GP Psychotherapist and a Senior Lecturer at the University of Queensland, Australia. She consults on family violence and neglect in primary care and teaches GPs and medical students in whole person care. She was recently awarded her PhD developing the concept of *sense of safety* as a whole person approach to distress.

Routledge Advances in the Medical Humanities

Reconsidering Dementia Narratives
Empathy, Identity and Care
Rebecca A. Bitenc

Moments of Rupture: The Importance of Affect in Surgical Training and Medical Education
Perspectives from Professional Learning and Philosophy
Arunthathi Mahendran

Storytelling Encounters as Medical Education
Crafting Relational Identity
Sally Warmington

Educating Doctors' Senses Through the Medical Humanities
'How Do I Look?'
Alan Bleakley

Medical Humanities, Sociology and the Suffering Self
Surviving Health
Wendy Lowe

A Whole Person Approach to Wellbeing
Building Sense of Safety
Johanna Lynch

Rethinking Pain in Person-Centred Health Care
Around Recovery
Stephen Buetow

Medical Education, Politics and Social Justice
The Contradiction Cure
Alan Bleakley

For more information about this series visit: www.routledge.com/Routledge-Advances-in-the-Medical-Humanities/book-series/RAMH

A Whole Person Approach to Wellbeing

Building Sense of Safety

Johanna Lynch

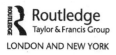
Routledge
Taylor & Francis Group

LONDON AND NEW YORK

First published 2021
by Routledge
2 Park Square, Milton Park, Abingdon, Oxon OX14 4RN

and by Routledge
52 Vanderbilt Avenue, New York, NY 10017

Routledge is an imprint of the Taylor & Francis Group, an informa business

British Library Cataloguing-in-Publication Data
A catalogue record for this book is available from the British Library

Library of Congress Cataloging-in-Publication Data
A catalog record has been requested for this book

ISBN: 978-0-367-49157-4 (hbk)
ISBN: 978-1-003-04483-3 (ebk)

Typeset in Times
by Deanta Global Publishing Services, Chennai, India

Contents

Figures

Tables

Foreword

Rarely do I receive a manuscript that excites me enough to not be able to put it down until the end and then spend days thinking about its implications, going back to sections to reread and rethink.

A Whole Person Approach to Wellbeing: Building Sense of Safety, from the PhD by Johanna Lynch, is one such book.

From the first line of the introduction, 'the beautiful, shiny, blue-black bird called the Satin Bowerbird as they gather what seems to be bits and pieces that attract them', we are alerted to something different. With the invitation to join the search for meaning in the whole story, the reader understands the critical need to see and come to know the whole person and the whole social system in which that person lives. And here is the challenge for workers within health care systems.

Although written from a general practitioner (GP's or family doctor's) perspective, this book has a strong message across all disciplines and systems.

Leading up to and during the time I was reading the draft, we were facing a number of crises in Australia and worldwide: the fires, floods and hail-storms in Australia, Coronavirus – COVID-19 – worldwide and Black Lives Matter moving from the United States of America and around the world. With what seemed like crisis after crisis, 'all the King's horses and all the King's men would never be able to put Humpy Dumpty back together again' unless we learn some lessons. Within this book there is a message for us all. The political leaders – 'all the King's Men' – cannot repair Humpy, so the prescription for building a *sense of safety* is a call to us all.

The 'permanent inquisitiveness' as a research approach and the 'disciplined self-reflexivity' as an essential contribution to who we are is vital as we find better ways of living together on this home we call earth. Hence, as I reread the book, I began thinking of not just ways to care for the whole person in medical practice but also as a way to care for the world as a whole. While attention is called to the whole person, aligning with the 1986 Ottawa Charter on health as 'peace, shelter, education, food, income, a stable eco-system, sustainable resources, social justice and equity', this is also a call to health within a whole ecosystem.

And this comes with a call to bring skills into focus for us all to 'adapt and self-manage in the face of social, physical and emotional challenges' in a rapidly changing world. So this is a prescription way beyond medicine.

But for this moment let us focus on the skills of a doctor to empower. Many years ago, I went to my GP with a continuing problem. He said he needed to refer me to a gynaecologist. Based on previous experiences, I was reluctant, and he said I should tell the gynaecologist of a childhood experience that I had shared with him. After an initial review of my medical records and small talk, the specialist asked me to 'get up on the couch'. I froze and then said I had something tell him. He looked up from writing on his records and stopped for a moment before putting his pen down and turning to face me, allowing me to sense he would listen beyond a general doctor's visit. I told him of the difficulty I have in such examinations and then related child harm of a sexual nature. He sat listening, attentive, fully present. Then he said quietly: 60 per cent of the women who need surgery in middle age have been sexually abused as a child. I was stunned, and then because of his manner, I felt empowered to ask him a question. Why have I not read about this in medical literature as I try to understand myself? His response was, 'because my colleagues do not see that is a relevant factor in their work [pause], but I think I need to take this discussion to our next meeting'. My GP empowered me, and because of that, the specialist decided to raise an issue for discussion at his next AGM. I felt heard. My *sense of safety* deepened not just with these two medical professionals but within myself as I grew in confidence to speak out.

This is a strengths-based approach to our professional relationships with me as a client of the doctors who respected my story as one of value to diagnosis and treatment.

While Johanna Lynch writes of mapping the *sense of safety* in whole person domains, Humpty's own capacity to attend to his own wounding is vital. If 'all the King's Men' can't repair Humpty, responsibility comes back to relationship – partnership – doctors and clients working together and perhaps Humpty doing some work as well.

Recently, in one workshop with medical and related health professionals, we asked participants to do either a genogram or a loss history map. The two people who were most impacted by the activity were doctors. One clearly saw a pattern across four generations within her family as she isolated herself from unresolved pain, moving, always moving, as had happened within each generation. The other, a male, saw in his deep inner reflection that he lectures clients about their drinking and each night he goes home and does exactly the same – drinks himself to sleep.

While the work of this book has not yet found its home because it is not covered by any specific single discipline, there is an indigenous epistemology and ontology which is very close to the theoretical transdisciplinary approach presented. There is perhaps a relationship between indigenous critical pedagogy and within indigenous healing practices.

This book is building a case for the concept of *sense of safety* as a central consideration in the relationship between client, practitioner and researcher as part of a whole.

Johanna Lynch wrote, we learn together, not just from Bowerbirds, but from wise clinicians, patients, stories and even from the Humpty Dumpty nursery rhyme. We learn as we listen to each, crossing pathways and disciplines and always as humans searching for that *sense of safety* in a world that is becoming increasingly unsafe. This book, *A Whole Person Approach to Wellbeing*, opens many doors and invites us to be, not King's Men, but wise learners as we listen to and learn from each other.

Judy Atkinson OAM PhD Emeritus Professor Southern Cross University Elder Advisor to We Al-Li (Culturally Informed Trauma Integrated Healing Training)

During the last five decades, we have witnessed the polarisation of two groups of Western biomedical professionals into two 'movements' holding fundamentally divergent points of view. One group enthusiastically welcomes the shift in clinical practice toward being ever more informed by technology, becoming more reliant on it, even being dominated by it. Others, meanwhile, particularly professionals in health care and population health care, have grown increasingly critical and outspoken about precisely that shift toward high-tech bio-medicine, which they perceive as nothing less than the institutionalisation of the dehumanisation of medicine.

These critical voices identified the dangers of medicalisation itself as it spread throughout all strata of every society. They began by demanding change at the core of each medical encounter, in what is traditionally referred to as the doctor-patient relationship. They called for the focus there to shift from being *medicine*-centred to being *patient*-centred. The dominant, medicine-centred gaze involves the physician observing her or his professional object, namely the patient. Implicit in such a gaze is not a mere objectification of the patient; it is a subordination.

Psychiatrist Georg Engel, the most influential voice early on in this critical development, proposed a much heralded and rapidly adopted 'model' termed the *biopsychosocial* approach to disease. While the intention was to encompass all those aspects of life that could be assumed to have an impact on health, it was never properly grounded theoretically. Engel and his colleagues neither elaborated on how to distinguish the 'biological', 'psychological' and 'social' aspects of human life from one another, nor, more crucially, on how to apply such distinctions to any specific patient's case. Each of these three disciplines has its own complex history and terminology; they could not be united by fiat, through a purely linguistic exercise of hyphenating them. Nor could the term *biopsychosocial* be applied within an actual medical practice – not intuitively, not functionally and certainly not automatically. Thus, despite being widely quoted and referred to, Engel's model remained a mere model.

It became clear to the proponents of the patient-centred approach that many in need of health care were inadequately served by the prevailing, strictly scientific, biological definition and classification of disease. Since any comprehensive understanding of an individual's suffering requires the integration of data about that patient's psychological and social conditions, they proposed broadening the scope of what to define as relevant patient information.

This acknowledgement of the general impact of life circumstances on health led to increased awareness of the crucial difference between a *patient* – which is a social role defined and assigned by medicine – and a *person* – which is a human being in her or his own right, bearing a world of personal experience complete with socio-cultural meaning. Physician and philosopher Eric Cassell advocated explicitly for *personhood* to be considered a relevant medical issue. This came to be mirrored in another and more recent shift from advocating *patient*-centred to *person*-centred medicine. This change also leaves out something essential, however: awareness of the fundamental reality that each medical encounter is a meeting of *two persons*, one in the role of patient, the other in the role of doctor, each of whom embodies an entire lifetime of experience.

The calls for such changes are not only anchored in a philosophically grounded defence of human integrity but also in a rapidly accumulating body of biomedical research; this documents the reality that human beings are affected, from the macro to the micro levels, by embodied, lived experience. The solid biomedical evidence that we now have about the detrimental impact that longstanding, burdensome adversity has on health enables us to conclude: the traditional schism within Western medicine has now been transcended. The human being's mind can no longer be seen as separate from the human being's body. Mind impacts on matter, even at the micro level. In short, mind matters.

That is what this book is about. It offers ways to understand not only *that* but also *how* mind matters and how subjective experience and lived meaning are established and embodied. The book is in part a response to Georg Engel's early critique of his own model. He amended his initial question, 'Is grief a disease?' and asked, instead: 'When is grief a disease?'

The author of this book would most probably answer Engel's decisive question this way: 'Unresolved grief is probably one of the deepest sources of disease since the experience of bereavement deprives you not only of a significant other but also of your equally consequential sense of dwelling safely in your life-world.'

Enriching the author's detailed reflections on the significance that a *sense of safety* holds for human beings are her personal reflections on how she herself has internalised personhood, what Cassell identified as every human being's existential ground. This inevitably involves being socialised into systems of symbols, rules and values, which are constituted inter-subjectively. One cannot simply step away from these 'webs of meaning', as anthropologist Clifford Geertz refers to them. An experienced general practitioner and therapist, Dr Lynch examines her own unique, cross-cultural situatedness, recognising it as a professional resource. She finds it creates a common ground, an experiential platform from which she is better able to see and understand the suffering of her fellow human beings.

Anna Luise Kirkengen, MD, PhD Professor in General Practice, NTNU Trondheim, Norway

Preface

As I approach the task of introducing this book and myself as author, I am drawn to a question that has inhabited and inspired my clinical and research work and this book. It is a central human question:

> What happens to states of mind when a sense of terror or grief is not met by reasonably attuned comforting?
>
> (Allen 2013, xiii)

What does happen to our whole beings, not just our minds, when we sense terror or grief? From our cells to our communities, what happens? Equally, what happens when we sense joy, belonging or safety?

This question names the processes I have observed in clinical practice as the honest people in my world have shown me their unmasked states of mind and fragmented, complex selves. They have taught me the raw beauty of sensing terror, sorrow and tuned-in, comforting connection in the presence of another person. Fundamentally, this question attends to the many people in our world who never receive 'reasonably attuned comforting' (Allen 2013, xiii). This book is for them.

There are all sorts of seemingly unsolvable reasons why people are 'uncomforted'. As a clinician, I believe the most fragile and unreasonable of these are medical and social science theories that propose themselves as adequate ways to assess distress and yet do not tune-in to the whole person's story or to evidence beyond their discipline. I write this book as a general practitioner (or family physician) who is tired of seeing people reduced by public discourse and diagnoses to simplistic medicalised stereotypes that often do not even acknowledge the existence of terror, grief, or comfort. I write in response to watching systemic fragmentation and narrowed dehumanising clinical realities for my patients, myself and my generalist colleagues. I write also as a generalist who has identified a pattern that I think may offer a way forward.

Robert Centor (2007, 59) declares 'to be a great physician you must understand the whole story ... gather the history at appropriate depth'. What is that whole story? What is an appropriate depth? These are generalist questions that all of us can ask as we search for ways to offer comfort and courage in our world.

As a clinician who sees patterns across the community – from schools, to workplaces, to healthcare settings – this book is a direct plea for a new way of attending to the whole person and defining appropriate depth. It is a plea for a shift from privileging narrow forms of evidence towards whole ways of seeing and understanding. Dividing the body and mind in order to carefully study or treat the person has created other forms of blindness. Despite intending to see the whole, these siloed approaches stop us seeing the person as a unified, interconnected and complex – a whole person who participates in and observes their own experience.

This book is a blueprint for a new unifying cross-cultural language which enables practitioners and the people they care for to see the whole story at an appropriate depth. It explains the value of wide ways of seeing the whole that no longer disconnect relationship and body, mind and meaning, community and physiology.

This book is written as a direct outworking of my own life story, cross-cultural skill set and generalist clinical work. I have spent my years as a generalist in the position of clinician near the social chaos of community, the 'non-expert' near the biotechnical or social science disciplinary experts. This has meant being 'out of my comfort zone' and being near others' jargon-filled 'certainty'. This place, on the border of disciplines and community, requires an attitude of cultural humility, curiosity, uncertainty and openness to connecting to other people and their ways of seeing the world. I have found others on this border-spanning journey – clinicians, researchers and friends across the globe who have given me the strength to ask perturbing questions and seek cross-disciplinary answers.

As an embedded participatory researcher, I introduce myself and my cross-cultural and transdisciplinary credentials: I was born in Belfast and grew up in Uganda. At age seven, my family fled dictator Idi Amin to Australia. My teen years were spent in Kenya, Australia and Indonesia before completing my medical training at The University of Queensland, Australia. Living life on the border – marked by skin colour, accent, culture and areas of knowledge that are incomplete has meant that I have spent my life trying to read unsaid clues and fragments of relevance in the dominant cultures around me. I have spent my life looking for patterns: for ways to understand, connect and belong. My migrant upbringing has prepared me for the transdisciplinary research and practice required to question medicine's established silos.

Searching for patterns and ways to care for the whole person in their community has been part of the 25 years I have spent as a general practitioner (family doctor). My work shifted in response to a need in my community, to care for those who often were told they had mental illness (and many other illnesses beside) but who actually were adult survivors of childhood trauma and neglect. This led to a search for clues to understand why their pain and its physical impacts (and the robust research in this area) had been largely ignored by modern medicine. I therefore shifted clinical practice and developed a transdisciplinary clinic called Integrate Place for five years, which included mental health nursing, social work, art and music therapies. Taking my biomedical training and the apprenticeship of my patients' stories, I searched for transdisciplinary approaches to whole person care through a program of doctoral research, presented in this book.

At the very beginning of my PhD thesis I was encouraged to write as though I was explaining my thesis question to a ten-year-old. The resulting poem presented below gives a hint of how this book may offer a map, a journey and a reason to travel towards more attuned comforting. This comfort requires a coherent language and unified way to see the whole person.

Is it possible
to work together
to see the big picture
of what helps people to live
their own lives well?

Is it possible
that something ordinary
but precious
might be really important
to see, and sustain?

A human
relational
necessity
that helps us
to grow?

This way of seeing might look
for people, places, perspectives
of security and capacity
to slowly find
the journey and the map.

Throughout this book, at times, I will refer to 'us' or 'we'– this is in deference to you the reader. I hope that you will journey with me as we progress together towards the robust conceptualisation of *sense of safety* as a way to offer comfort and build wellbeing. I hope the insights in this book will give you tools to build your own *sense of safety* in the whole story of your personal and professional life and for those you research, care for and teach.

The ideas presented here are grounded in generalist clinical practice and transdisciplinary thinking; in respect for indigenous ways of knowing and relating; in learning from spiritual communities that value accurate but humble interpreting of context and meaning (hermeneutics) and in deference to those thinkers who wrote before the disciplines became established silos. These ideas are grounded in both academic and relational multidisciplinary learning in peer review groups (Living Wholeness and Integrate Place) over the last fifteen years. They are indebted to medical generalist physicians, paediatricians, family doctors and other physicians who have taught me to see the whole. They are influenced by people from other generalist professions – including teaching, nursing, social work, pastoral care and occupational therapy. They are fine-tuned by teaching medical students and general practitioners. Ultimately, these ideas are grounded in the bravery of my patients who revealed the patterns of their life stories, relationships and embodied experiences to me. They have encouraged me to value the wide view of the generalist. They have taught me the importance of safety. They have shown me the value of attuned comforting. They have encouraged me as they walked towards healing.

References

Allen, J. G. 2013. *Restoring mentalizing in attachment relationships: Treating trauma with plain old therapy.* Washington: American Psychiatric Publishing.

Centor, Robert M. 2007. 'To be a great physician, you must understand the whole story.' *Medscape General Medicine* 9 (1):59.

Acknowledgements

This book is dedicated to my husband Jim and children Kelsey, Rebekah and Matthew who make it safe for me to belong to them and continue to teach me about comfort and courage. Thank for helping me to keep in mind the deeper spiritual vision of safe refuge for our community, and thanks for the joy you are to me.

Thanks too to Megan Connell, Dawn Courtman and Pat Bryden, and wider family and friends who have walked this road with me.

In my professional life I owe a debt of gratitude to my patients who have taught me to see them and hear their lived and embodied experience, who inspired this work and who encouraged me to continue to search for *sense of safety* in their lives, my own life and in the writings and research of others.

Thank you to the teams at A Place to Belong, Blue Knot foundation and the Australian Society for Psychological Medicine who have encouraged me and those at Zest Infusion who have supported my clinical work during this time. Thank you too to the team at Routledge who have made turning it into a book possible – especially Grace McInnes and Evie Lonsdale.

Another joy has been meeting mentors and thinkers who have been on this journey ahead of me and have generously included me. I offer thanks to my supervisors Professors Chris Dowrick, Mieke van Driel and Pamela Meredith who took a risk and invested in me and my PhD examiners Professors Kurt Stange and Linn Getz who encouraged me to keep going. I thank Professor Anna Luise Kirkengen who has given me the privilege of her thoughtful critique of a number of iterations of this book and the PhD that preceded it. Other key mentors along the journey have been Joanne Reeve, Robert Neimeyer, Martin Dorahy, Judith Murray, Geoff Mitchell, Judy Atkinson, Robert Maunder, William Miller, Carolyn Russell, Rachel Collis, Sue Hooper, John Warlow, Paul Mercer, Andrew Wright, Margaret Kay, Maree Toombs, Joe Tucci, Michaela Kelly, Deb Askew, Sue McGregor, Cathy Kezelman, Pam Stravropoulos, Jon Hunter, May-Lill Johansen, Jayne Ingham, Mary Emeleus, Deb Weins, Chris Bauer, Hugh Norriss, Jenny Brown, Natasha Rae, Ken Kunin and Kay Hooper. I also thank Vicki Binnie, Susan Coutts, Fiona Stevens, Karen Misso, Karen Liddle, Andy Pocock, Ashley Withers, Peter Hayton and Jono Andrews from the Integrate Place and Living Wholeness multidisciplinary peer support groups. Thank you for steadying me, refining the ideas and investing your time into this endeavour.

Introduction

In the Australian rainforest near my home there is a beautiful shiny blue-black bird called the Satin Bowerbird. This bird spends its life collecting blue pen and milk bottle lids, straws and fragments of blue foil and brings them home to decorate his bower. He searches and searches for blue things and brings each disparate object back faithfully, instinctively. When viewed from a distance, his pedantic obsessive search for useless bits of plastic has somehow gathered into a beautiful pattern. The Bowerbird has not just been gathering randomly; he has been carefully choosing and placing each part of what becomes a whole.

The Bowerbird's gathering involves decisions about what scope and depth of search is appropriate, how to discern what is valuable and how to hold them together. These are sophisticated skills that can often appear simple (or inexpert) if done well. This gathering is the task of anyone who seeks to attend to and care for a whole person.

Seeing the whole is not easy. The myriad of possible physical, psychological, social, spiritual or environmental causes of distress can be overwhelming (Dowrick 2004). Whether in family or work dynamics, in attempts to understand our friends or those we disagree with, or in practical decisions in schools, workplaces and healthcare, seeing the whole is hard work. Yet it is so necessary.

There are many factors that can get in the way of seeing the whole person. There are philosophical, political, professional and financial forces beyond the scope of this book that contribute to good science being ignored, to parts of the whole being side-lined, to an incoherence and confusion that blinds us to the whole. When facing the insular prejudice of his profession as he investigated the link between family violence and psychopathology, John Bowlby (1984, 9) reported: 'it has been extremely unfashionable to attribute psychopathology to real-life experiences'. In the realm of science, what does fashion have to do with it? Fashions can help us to see paradigms that influence what is seen (and not seen) and how it is valued (or devalued).

This book is unashamedly generalist in its viewpoint. As we progress together, I hope you will be convinced of the unique transdisciplinary gifts the generalist can offer to a world that has become fragmented. Seeing the whole person is a mindset that transcends disciplinary boundaries. This generalist mindset includes attitudes to the task of knowing, to tuning in, to defining the direction and purpose of care, to relationship and how subjective information is valued and to what is considered adequate breadth of scope. It can inhabit the way that anyone from any discipline tunes in to the people they are with, alongside their technical skills. For some professions, such as family medicine, palliative care, geriatrics, paediatrics, nursing, social work, occupational therapy and teaching, seeing the whole person is a fundamental part of practice.

The insights in this book are drawn from my medical training, clinical experience with patients and learning from multidisciplinary colleagues and extensive stakeholder and academic consultation across the disciplines as part of my doctoral research.[1] This research is indebted to those who wrote before the disciplines became well-established, those who have described and defended generalism and those who connect the biomedical and social science disciplines in transdisciplinary research and practice. In this book I will build on the wisdom of many general practitioners who have described, defined and defended generalism in the primary care setting (Gunn et al. 2008, Reeve 2010, Dowrick 2017, Stange 2009, Epstein 2013, Hutchinson 2011, Getz, Nilsson, and Hetlevik 2003, Heath 1997, McWhinney 1969, Rudebeck 2019, Pellegrino 1966).

Although the priority of whole person care has come from the generalist primary healthcare setting (Reeve et al. 2013), it is endorsed by transdisciplinary philosophy and research and by calls for change from other generalist fields (Muller 2018). The ideas presented in this book are relevant across our community.

This book is about shifting our mindsets and our hearts. It is written for academics, clinicians, educators, employers and leaders across the disciplines who recognise the complexity involved in seeing the whole and seek to refine their skills. It is written for all practitioners who seek overarching first principles to help them navigate siloed approaches to wellbeing. As we consider what fragments and insights to bring to the bower of whole person care, we will look through the wide, relational lens of the generalist. Attending to the whole through the philosophy, practice and language of generalism is relevant to any practitioner from education to healthcare who seeks to care for the whole person. What matters is seeing the whole person through the fragments and maintaining a focus on the beauty gathered in the bower.

Looking wide for the whole: The generalist gaze

The wide view of health described in this book aligns with the broad definition adopted by the World Health Organisation in 1948: 'A state of complete physical, mental and social well-being and not merely the absence of disease or infirmity' (WHO 2006). It also agrees with those who question the possibility of 'complete' well-being – instead calling for an understanding of health as the 'ability to adapt and self-manage in the face of social, physical and emotional challenges' (Huber et al. 2011, 343). The breadth of attention to the whole person also aligns with the conditions named in the 1986 Ottawa Charter as resources for health: peace, shelter, education, food, income, a stable eco-system, sustainable resources, social justice and equity.

In caring for this whole, practitioners need the Bowerbird's attitudes – to be open and willing to find the fragments and gather them together. Transdisciplinary researchers describe this as 'permanent inquisitiveness' (Augsburg 2014, 236), an openness, a creativity, 'a humble attitude towards the immensity of knowledge', 'disciplined self-reflexivity' and a capacity to resist being the 'alpha expert' (Augsburg 2014, McGregor 2015, McGregor and Donnelly 2014). Generalists describe the Bowerbird skill of gathering as 'inductive foraging' (Donner-Banzhoff and Hertwig 2014, 69), a process that values a broad view and cares for the whole person. The theme of 'looking wide' will be revisited often during this book, looking at the breadth of knowledge considered valid, at the practical skills of how to integrate and interpret knowledge and at the careful use of language that helps us see the whole. This wide view enables early pattern recognition and early intervention and also protects practitioners from what GPs call premature categorisation.

Using language that does not divide

The focus of this book is the person–resisting the draw to narrow the focus onto any particular body part or disorder. This includes resistance to using language that narrows or inadvertently aligns with dividing the whole (for example, dualist division into 'mind' and 'body'); jargon words that name things as though they are real entities separate to the whole (such as 'mental health' or 'psychopathology') or language that has become a shorthand caricature or stereotype that is no longer helpful for understanding the whole (such as 'anxious' or 'depressed'). As observant novelist Chimamanda Ngozi Adichie points out, these narrower words are incomplete: 'The problem with stereotypes is not that they are untrue, but they are incomplete, they make one story become the only story' (Adichie 2009).

Instead, the language in this book is wide and inclusive of complex multi-layered stories. It includes words that challenge us to keep our attention on the *whole person* who experiences *distress* and *threat*, and who seeks *healing* and *wellbeing*. These wide words set the scene and prevent narrowed views – they direct attention and perspective to notice the edges and include the variations. These ordinary non-jargon words facilitate a wide view for all involved. They set the scene for the wide stakeholder consultation and the search for a common transdisciplinary language that underpins this book.

This wide gaze will attend to the *whole person*. Although, the term 'person' is in itself a complex multi-layered whole, the term 'whole person' is used throughout this book to name an alternative to the paradigms and processes that fragment or simplify an understanding of personhood. Persons are made up of aspects or parts that need to be intentionally gathered so they can be cared for as a whole. The term 'whole person care' is used in preference to the terms 'patient or person-centred care' that may not include acknowledgement of physiology or the contextual and relational aspects of the personhood of both practitioner and distressed person (Dahlberg, Todres, and Galvin 2009).

Distress is a non-medical term describing an ordinary human experience that is encountered in any field of practice and is not always pathological. Use of this term points towards ordinary language and ways of understanding ill-health, 'unease' (Tomasdottir et al. 2016) or disheartening and discomforting life experiences. Distress – from the Latin *distringere* (to 'stretch apart') – could help us to understand how pain fragments. This approach helps the generalist to attend to the person who presents in undifferentiated distress. It widens our gaze to see the whole.

Distress is also a subjective experience that cannot be quantified by an external observer and therefore gives voice and self-definition to the sufferer – not an ascendant medical observer (Verhaeghe 2004). Distress also includes co-occurring phenomenon often referred to as 'comorbid' or 'multi-morbid' that may be considered (and studied) as separate pathological processes and yet occur within the same person at the same time, often more frequently than would be predicted by chance (Kirkengen 2018). It includes distress reduction behaviours or ways humans cope, such as many forms of addiction, obsessions, compulsions, phobias, suicidality and deliberate self-harm, as well as other defences such as workaholism or perfectionism that may mask underlying distress. The term 'distress' in this book includes normal responses to life experience such as grief, insomnia, agitated behaviours, violence, conflict, suffering, loss of concentration, pain, shame, regret, hopelessness and flashbacks (Epstein and Back 2015). It includes vague constellations of somatic complaints and other Medically Unexplained Symptoms (MUS), what some call somatoform disorders, and acute or chronic medical diagnoses. It includes the concepts of mental, psychological, bodily, existential, social, relational, environmental and even intergenerational distress as part of the whole person's experience.

Attending to *threat* is a way to attend to the many ways that people become distressed. 'What causes threat?' was a key research question to participants in my doctoral research to be discussed in later chapters. Abraham Maslow described the impact of threat on the 'whole human being … never a part of a human being' (Maslow 1954, 75).[2] He also noted the experience of overwhelm (and loss of capacity to cope with threat) as a process that caused the organism to 'disintegrate' (Maslow 1954, 11). In her work, Anna Luise Kirkengen, a GP researcher, describes the 'lived body' and declares that violation of integrity impacts health (Kirkengen and Thornquist 2012). There is also an implicit wide view of threat and its impact on integrity of the person in this description of suffering: 'Suffering occurs with perceived threat of destruction and ends when the threat has passed, or a sense of integrity is otherwise restored' (Mount, Boston, and Cohen 2007, 373).

Again, in order to preserve a wide perspective, generalists keep the end-goal in mind: *healing and wellbeing*. Instead of a focus on one aberration, or disease process, a focus on wellbeing and healing allows a range of distress to be attended to with a clear purpose. Healing is an active personal growth process. Palliative care physician, Balfour Mount, defines health as: the 'ability of people to move from suffering to a sense of integrity and wholeness often independent of objective improvement' (Hutchinson 2011, 1). *Wellbeing* is multifaceted – the word 'being' represents the whole organism as well as the dynamic whole person experience of 'being alive'. Christopher Dowrick (2009, 1146), a GP researcher, describes this core value of primary care as 'attempts to enable patients to engage or reengage with their lives as social beings'.

Attention to healing shifts the focus away from biotechnical cure towards relational healing connections. It offers a view of health as more than technoscientific (Vogt, Hofmann, and Getz 2016), as more than medicalisation and as able to encounter healing in the face of disease and even death. This humanistic or dignity-based view of health (Bleakley 2015, Marcum 2008, Jacobson 2007) will draw 'attention to wholeness, health and human life stories' (Vogt, Hofmann, and Getz 2016, 314).

Healing also includes the experience of being comforted or consoled. Hippocrates is credited with naming the goal of medicine as 'to cure sometimes, heal often and console always' (Ghaemi 2009, 4). The task of offering consolation is at the centre of the concept of *sense of safety* to be developed in this book. This concept of healing-oriented care offers a wide view of the person as more than bodily symptoms to be cured.

Although some thinkers critique the search for metanarratives or theoretical integration of parts (Lyotard 1984), others remind us: 'human experiences, and thus more generally human nature, are stable enough to make at least some provisional generalisations about them' (Low 2010, 199). Bradley Lewis (2014, 196) encourages us to 'develop better, truer, richer, more generous stories and case formulations in the service of healing and coping'. This is one of the goals of the new transdisciplinary language of *sense of safety* developed throughout this book. Perhaps movement from the threat inherent in distress and suffering towards healing can be achieved through facilitating and supporting (or *building*) a person's '*sense of safety*'.

The wide view of the *person*, their *distress* and their *healing* proposed in this book is offered to practitioners across the disciplines in the hope of changing mindsets and of encouraging research and practice that unites us in service of each person in distress. At times, the evidence presented in this book will be overly inclusive or extensively referenced in the hopes that you can take the breadth and validity of fragments gathered and apply them to your own discipline. I am hopeful they will be sufficient to convince you to lay a foundation for a new mindset about wellbeing wherever you belong.

Philosopher John Sadler (2005, 7) describes those who offer whole person care as 'beleaguered defender[s] of holism, empathy and the complex understanding of the individual'. I invite beleaguered defenders from every walk of life to come on a journey in this book as we learn together, not just from Bowerbirds, but from wise clinicians, researchers, patients, stories and even from the Humpty Dumpty nursery rhyme. We will learn how to see the whole, discern value and gather at appropriate depth. We will explore the potential for a new language – *sense of safety* – that might assist to unify scientific research and cross-disciplinary thinking and practice. We will search together for ways to see the whole person that will apply to practitioners in many parts of our communities worldwide

- This book is structured in two sections. The first section includes an overview of the philosophical and practical underpinnings of a whole person framework and justifies the decision to proceed to explore the use of the ordinary phrase 'sense of safety'
- The second section reports on the findings of this exploration and describes the conceptualisation of **sense of safety** – defining its domains and dynamics relevant to all people: researchers, practitioners and the wider community
- The term 'practitioner' (rather than 'clinician') is used throughout to clearly include generalists across the community beyond the medical or primary care sphere
- At times my doctoral research stakeholders will be referenced in the text: general practitioners (gp), patients (those with lived experience of being a patient — le), indigenous academics (ia) and multidisciplinary mental health clinicians (mhc)
- Doctoral consultation also included two reviews by a ten-member international multidisciplinary academic panel (denoted as mhc-a, and gp-a)

Notes

1 This book is based on my doctoral thesis, *Sense of safety: a whole person approach to distress*, conferred in September 2019 through the University of Queensland. This doctoral program of research was undertaken within the Primary Care Clinical Unit in the Faculty of Medicine. It was funded through the Australian Government and Advance Queensland Scholar programs and given ethical approval through the School of Medicine Low Risk Ethical Review Committee (2017-SOMILRE-0191). Stakeholders included in this focus group and interview consultation included two indigenous academics, 10 GPs, 20 mental health clinicians and nine people with a lived experience of being a patient.
2 Maslow named the threat to basic needs that comes from loss of freedom to speak, to express oneself, to seek information and to defend oneself (Maslow 1987). He named loss of 'justice, fairness, honesty and orderliness [and the existence of] secrecy, censorship, dishonesty and blocking of communication' as threats to basic needs (Maslow 1987, 22). Of course his hierarchy of needs, as will be discussed in Chapter Four, also named a range of causes of threat – across physiology, safety (by which he meant security, stability, protection, freedom from fear), belongingness and love, esteem and self-actualisation (Maslow 1987, 22).

References

Adichie, Chimamanda Ngozi. 2009. *The danger of a single story*. TED Talk. http://www.ted.com/talks/chimamanda_adichie_the_danger_of_a_single_story.html

Augsburg, Tanya. 2014. 'Becoming transdisciplinary: The emergence of the transdisciplinary individual.' *World Futures* 70 (3–4):233–247.

Bleakley, Alan. 2015. *Medical humanities and medical education: How the medical humanities can shape better doctors*. New York: Routledge.

Bowlby, J. 1984. 'Violence in the family as a disorder of the attachment and caregiving system.' *American Journal of Psychoanalysis* 44:9–27.

Dahlberg, Karin, Les Todres, and Kathleen Galvin. 2009. 'Lifeworld-led healthcare is more than patient-led care: An existential view of well-being.' *Medicine, Health Care and Philosophy* 12 (3):265–271.

Donner-Banzhoff, Norbert, and Ralph Hertwig. 2014. 'Inductive foraging: Improving the diagnostic yield of primary care consultations.' *The European Journal of General Practice* 20 (1):69–73.

Dowrick, Christopher. 2004. *Beyond depression: A new approach to understanding and management*. London: Oxford University Press.

Dowrick, Christopher. 2009. 'When diagnosis fails: A commentary on McPherson & Armstrong.' *Social Science & Medicine* 69 (8):1144–1146.

Dowrick, Christopher. 2017. *Person-centred primary care: Searching for the self*. London: Routledge.

Epstein, Ronald Mark, and Anthony L. Back. 2015. 'Responding to suffering.' *JAMA* 314 (24):2623–2624.

Epstein, Ronald Mark. 2013. 'Whole mind and shared mind in clinical decision-making.' *Patient Education and Counseling* 90 (2):200–206.

Getz, Linn, Peter M. Nilsson, and Irene Hetlevik. 2003. 'A matter of heart: The general practitioner consultation in an evidence-based world.' *Scandinavian Journal of Primary Health Care* 21 (1):3–9.

Ghaemi, S.N. 2009. 'Nosologomania: DSM & Karl Jaspers' critique of Kraepelin.' *Philosophy, Ethics, and Humanities in Medicine* 4 (1):10. https://doi.org/10.1186/1747-5341-4-10.

Gunn, J.M., V.J. Palmer, L. Naccarella, R. Kokanovic, C.J. Pope, J. Lathlean, and K. Stange. 2008. 'The promise and pitfalls of generalism in achieving the Alma-Ata vision of health for all.' *Medical Journal of Australia* 189 (2):110–112.

Heath, I., ed. 1997. *The mystery of general practice*. London: Nuffield Provincial Hospital Trust.

Huber, Machteld, J. André Knottnerus, Lawrence Green, Henriëtte van der Horst, Alejandro R. Jadad, Daan Kromhout, Brian Leonard, Kate Lorig, Maria Isabel Loureiro, and Jos W.M. van der Meer. 2011. 'How should we define health?' *BMJ* 343:d4163. doi:10.1136/bmj.d4163

Hutchinson, T.A. 2011. *Whole person care: A new paradigm for the 21st century*. New York: Springer.

Jacobson, Nora. 2007. 'Dignity and health: A review.' *Social Science & Medicine* 64 (2):292–302.

Kirkengen, Anna Luise. 2018. 'From wholes to fragments to wholes – what gets lost in translation?' *Journal of Evaluation in Clinical Practice* 24 (5):1145–1149.

Kirkengen, Anna Luise, and Eline Thornquist. 2012. 'The lived body as a medical topic: An argument for an ethically informed epistemology.' *Journal of Evaluation in Clinical Practice* 18 (5):1095–1101.

Lewis, Bradley. 2014. 'The four Ps, narrative psychiatry, and the story of George Engel.' *Philosophy, Psychiatry, & Psychology* 21 (3):195–197.

Low, Douglas. 2010. 'Merleau-Ponty and a reconsideration of alienation.' *Philosophy Today* 54 (2):199–211.

Lyotard, Jean-François. 1984. *The postmodern condition: A report on knowledge*. Vol. 10. Minneapolis: University of Minnesota Press.

Marcum, James A. 2008. *Humanizing modern medicine: An introductory philosophy of medicine*. Edited by S.F. Spicker, H.T. Engelhardt, and L.M. Rasmussen. Vol. 99, Philosophy and medicine. Baylor University: Springer.

Maslow, A.H. 1987. *Motivation and personality third edition*. Edited by R. Frager, J. Fadiman, C. McReynolds, and R. Cox. New York: Harper Collins Publishers.

Maslow, A.H. 1954. *Motivation and personality third edition*. Edited by R. Frager, J. Fadiman, C. McReynolds, and R. Cox New York: Harper Collins Publishers.

McGregor, S.L.T. 2015. 'Transdisciplinary knowledge creation.' In *Transdisciplinary professional learning and practice*, edited by P. Gibbs, 9–24. New York: Springer.

McGregor, S.L.T., and Gabrielle Donnelly. 2014. 'Transleadership for transdisciplinary initiatives.' *World Futures* 70 (3–4):164–185.

McWhinney, Ian R. 1969. 'The foundations of family medicine.' *Canadian Family Physician* 15 (4):13–27.

Mount, Balfour M., Patricia H. Boston, and S. Robin Cohen. 2007. 'Healing connections: On moving from suffering to a sense of well-being.' *Journal of Pain and Symptom Management* 33 (4):372–388.

Muller, Jerry Z. 2018. *The tyranny of metrics*: Princeton: Princeton University Press.

Pellegrino, Edmund D. 1966. 'The generalist function in medicine.' *JAMA* 198 (5):541–545.

Reeve, J. 2010. 'Interpretive medicine: Supporting generalism in a changing primary care world.' *Occasional Paper Royal College of General Practitioners* 88:1–20.

Reeve, J., C. Dowrick, F.G.K. Freeman, J. Gunn, F. Mair, C. May, S. Mercer, V. Palmer, A. Howe, and G. Irving. 2013. 'Examining the practice of generalist expertise: A qualitative study identifying constraints and solutions.' *JRSM Short Reports* 4 (12):1–9.

Rudebeck, Carl Edvard. 2019. 'Relationship based care–how general practice developed and why it is undermined within contemporary healthcare systems.' *Scandinavian Journal of Primary Health Care* 37 (3):335–344.

Sadler, J.Z. 2005. *Values and psychiatric diagnosis*. Oxford: Oxford University Press.

Stange, Kurt C. 2009. 'The generalist approach.' *The Annals of Family Medicine* 7 (3):198–203.

Tomasdottir, Margret Olafia, Johann Agust Sigurdsson, Halfdan Petursson, Anna Luise Kirkengen, Tom Ivar Lund Nilsen, Irene Hetlevik, and Linn Getz. 2016. 'Does 'existential unease' predict adult multimorbidity? Analytical cohort study on embodiment based on the Norwegian HUNT population.' *BMJ Open* 6 (11):e012602. doi:10.1136/bmjopen-2016-012602.

Verhaeghe, Paul, ed. 2004. *On being normal and other disorders: A manual for clinical psychodiagnostics*. New York: Other Press.

Vogt, Henrik, Bjørn Hofmann, and Linn Getz. 2016. 'The new holism: P4 systems medicine and the medicalization of health and life itself.' *Medicine, Health Care and Philosophy* 19 (2):307–323.

WHO. 2006. *Constitution of the World Health Organization*. World Health Organisation. (30 June 2011; http://www.who.int/governance/eb/who_constitution_en.pdf).

Section One

Building a case for a shift in practitioner and researcher mindset

John Sadler (2005, 7), a medical philosopher, warns: "the way a question is posed constrains the possible answers". This section progressively builds an argument for generalist scope, transdisciplinary philosophy, senses as integrative and safety as essential for wellbeing.

Building over five chapters, this argument at times calls on the metaphor of Humpty Dumpty as a way to conceptualise a whole that can be seen in parts that the King's Men (those who care for and research Humpty) find difficult to bring back together. This clinical, theoretical and scientific discussion lays the foundation for new questions. Section One is designed to shift our mindset so we might be open to the new answers presented in Section Two. Section One builds a case that is made practical in Section Two, suggesting new questions that might offer new answers to how wellbeing is conceptualised across our community.

Reference

Sadler, J. Z. 2005. *Values and psychiatric diagnosis*. Oxford: Oxford University Press.

1 Transcending parts to see a whole – Humpty Dumpty represents us all

- Humpty Dumpty, the nursery rhyme character, is a metaphoric representation of all people
- Generalist and transdisciplinary approaches include a wide scope, relational process, healing purpose and integrative wisdom in order to see the whole
- The Aboriginal concept of 'Dadirri' can enrich our understanding of the whole
- It matters that the language we use reminds us to look wide

Years ago, a patient, 'Linda', asked me a haunting question:

> I've lived my life in this hole. Why did it take so long? No one was looking for what you were looking for.

When I look at these words, I can see that when Linda described being 'in a hole' she was unable to see herself as a whole. Why did it take so long? Why was no one looking? Linda had been seen by teachers, employers, psychiatrists, inpatient mental health teams, dieticians, psychologists and other family doctors over the years. Care and help could have come to Linda when she was a child, or during her violent marriage – sometime before her children were grown up, before she started to not care about her weight or her life. Instead, a focus on symptoms and deficits and biomedical priorities fragmented how Linda was seen. Linda also found it difficult to see her whole self – she experienced internal scattering of attention and altered perceptions of her body and relationships. Internal and external narrowed attention made it harder to get out of the 'hole'.

Later in Linda's story we discovered together that in her teens she had dreamt of learning to deep sea kayak. Acting on this dream gave her hours of pleasure, sources of good seafood and healthy weight loss. She was able to wean off high-dose antidepressants and mood stabilisers and reclaim her role as mother in her family. Linda's words and her story have impacted my research and clinical work. They have led me to ask new questions about what we should be looking for in order to see the whole. What if seeing the whole is a prerequisite for creativity, connection and a sense of humour? What if seeing the whole makes it possible to see unexpected possibilities for healing and growth? Maybe siloed medicine is missing something – leaving fragments out of the bower, and not noticing patterns of the whole that could help people like Linda. Perhaps siloed medicine cannot be considered compassionate, personalised, moral or scientifically accurate if it does not see the whole person and intentionally help them out of their 'hole'.

The centrality of personhood to whole person care

When I teach medical students about whole person care, I use the nursery rhyme character of Humpty Dumpty[1] to symbolise a whole person. Medical students can relate to the idea of fragmented medicine and understand the need to remember that Humpty was a complex, multilayered whole before he[2] fell. Humpty could symbolise a patient,[3] a student, an employee, a client, a workmate or a family member – a person across different settings. And, of course, Humpty also represents the clinician, teacher, policy writer, employer or leader – each type of practitioner.[4]

Humpty is not just 'disembodied genes, minds, and behaviours' (Krieger 2005, 351) but a complex embodied social being and biological organism. Humpty represents this whole self, embedded in community, history and environment, who can tell us verbal and embodied stories. Linn Getz, a GP researcher (2011, 1), reminds us of the need to acknowledge the 'self-aware, meaning-making, purposeful and relational nature of humans [and be aware of] how experiences associated with self-image, relations and values become inscribed in the body'. To know Humpty as a whole person requires a capacity to see objectively and listen subjectively to discern what is going on. It could even be argued that a commitment to this whole-hearted relational process of seeing, listening, questioning and discerning is an act of justice (Fricker 2007; Lynch, 2020).

A key assumption that underlies whole person care is the inherent value, agency, subjective sense of self, sacred dignity and lived experience of each person. Eric Cassell (2010, 50) describes a person as:

> an embodied, purposeful, thinking, feeling, emotional, reflective, relational, human individual always in action, responsive to meaning, and whose life in all spheres points both outward and inward. Virtually all of a person's actions – volitional, habitual, instinctual, or automatic – are based on meanings. Persons live at all times in a context of ever present relationships in which a variable degree of trust is necessary both in others and in the self.

Central to this definition is an awareness of the contextual, meaningful and relational aspects of the person and the responsive inward and outward dynamics of the person. Importantly, as we consider threat later in this book, the impact of threat on the person is implied in the phrase 'variable degree of trust'. It is this complex relational, active, reflective person who Humpty represents.

In her thorough treatise on generalism as an interpretive approach to knowledge in a clinical encounter, Joanne Reeve (2010), a GP researcher, reminds us that, in order to offer patient-centred holistic care, general practitioners need to integrate different sources of knowledge, including the voice of the patient. Kirkengen (2005, 20) calls us to notice 'the lives, hopes, intentions, defeats and longings of our patients – respectfully'. While Maslow (1954, 195) names the intentional effort of this task 'whole-hearted attending':

> Categorising is definitely less fatiguing than whole-hearted attending ... it does not call for concentration, it does not demand all the resources of the organism.

Whole-hearted attending: How to walk the journey with Humpty

So, how do generalists integrate these ways of knowing? How do they gather knowledge, sift it for usefulness and work out what is most important? In the language of the Bowerbird, how do they decide what fragments to bring home? The philosophical, intellectual and practical aspects of these skills organise and prioritise attention and perception. For the generalist, practical wisdom (*phronesis*) needs to be valued alongside knowledge (*episteme*) and skills (*techne*) (Epstein 2014).

The following definition of generalism will be used to define the scope of whole person care in this book:

> A professional philosophy of healthcare practice described as 'expertise in whole person medicine'. The 'expertise' of generalism relates to an approach to care which is person not disease oriented; taking a continuous rather than an episodic view; integrating biomedical and biographical understanding of illness; to support decisions which recognise health as a resource for living and not an end in itself.
>
> (Reeve et al. 2013, 1)

This inclusion of biology *and* biography (or life story) offers an antidote to the biotechnical knowledge silos of our age that Donald Schön (1995) calls 'technical reductionism'. Described further as a craft – generalist principles can be distilled to include 'whole person scope', 'relational process', 'healing purpose' and 'integrative wisdom' (see Figure 1.1) (Lynch 2019, Lynch et al. 2020).

Transdisciplinary philosophy and practice align with generalism and can be considered an epistemology – Transdisciplinary Generalism (Lynch et al. 2020). This underpins the approach to the whole person outlined in this book. Transdisciplinarity is:

> a perspective, engagement and action that is at once between the disciplines, across the different disciplines, and beyond each individual discipline. Its goal is the understanding of the present world from different perspectives (or

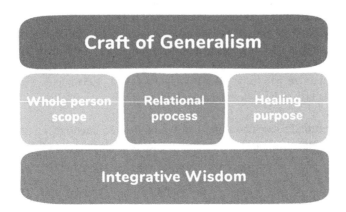

Figure 1.1 The *craft of generalism.*

realities), of which one of the imperatives is the overarching unity of knowledge through integration.

(McIntosh, Jeffery, and Muhajarine 2010, xviii)

Transdisciplinarity requires a cultural humility that values forms of knowledge across the disciplines and is not satisfied with simplistic categorisations or labelling of Humpty. This broad vision values both certainty and uncertainty, observation as well as participation, inductive and deductive reasoning, linear reason as well as complexity, and a capacity to reflect and integrate. Seeing the whole person involves relationship, a focus on healing-centred goals, and the use of integrative skills that require wisdom.

Relational process: 'Being with' the person

The time spent building a relationship with Humpty is a key part of whole person care. The task of attending to the whole person is undertaken within trusting, attuned, respectful relationships that turn towards suffering (Epstein and Back 2015). 'Being with' assumes interviewing and 'outerviewing', as well as communing, communicating and sensuous knowing (Reason and Bradbury 2001, 12, Epstein 2014, 277). These relational processes include what generalists name 'shared presence' (Ventres and Frankel 2015),[5] 'dogged determination to see through the patient's eyes' (Allen 2013, xii), collaborative deliberation (Popa, Guillermin, and Dedeurwaerdere 2015, Elwyn et al. 2014) and 'abiding … a promise not to abandon the patient even if pills and technology have little left to offer' (Scott et al. 2008). Transdisciplinary researchers describe this process as a 'working alliance' (Gray 2008, S126) or 'mutual learning' (Carew and Wickson 2010, 1148).

Australian Aboriginal people use the term 'Dadirri'[6] to communicate a 'shared dialogue … [a] deep contemplative process of 'listening to one another' in reciprocal relationship' (Ungunmerr 1993, Atkinson 2002, 15). These relationships offer safety (Atkinson 2002) and listening that 'invites responsibility to get the story – the information – right' (Atkinson 2002, 18) and requires 'mind-heart connection' (Atkinson 2002, 19). Dadirri also considers community and reciprocity in each interaction, searching for deep meaning and understanding. Similarly, general practitioners, due to their long-standing relationships with people over time, can build trust in a way that leads patients to say: 'I've never told anyone else, but …'. This sort of relationship can enable the disclosure of information often hidden from others, facilitating more accurate understanding (Epstein 2014). Disclosure in the context of safe relationships is a necessary prerequisite for accurate seeing of the whole.

Healing orientation: Clarity about why knowledge is gathered

Healing-oriented care is an important way that generalists manage attention to the whole. Keeping a focus on the goal of care provides an effective way to include the many complex factors that can impact wellbeing. If a general practitioner knows what constitutes a healthy blood pressure, they can attend to any change in blood pressure (hypo or hypertension) and can be open to the many processes that impact blood pressure (e.g., renal disease, endocrine dysfunction, lung fibrosis, dehydration or myocardial hypertrophy or failure, or even salt intake). A clinician who has a broad focus on the whole person will attend to anything that threatens that healing goal. They will be aware of threat or resources – patterns that change or support that wellbeing goal – from physical to subjective or even existential sources.

As mentioned earlier, a wide goal of healing attends to the needs of the whole person and not just a part. Bodily symptoms, addictions, work performance or school grades are just a part of a life filled with dreams and hopes, fears and wishes, relationships and meaning. In the face of complex illness and life stories, a focus on healing establishes priorities for the gathering of knowledge. This process takes us beyond behaviours or the symptoms and disease identification of cure-based medicine and toward meaning, relationships and a sense of self. If Humpty and his carers have a joint understanding of these healing goals, they will direct attention towards identifying the strengths and resources available that support adapting, growing and enablement (Howie et al. 1998). An essential aspect of this process involves the goal of facilitating the person to become 'safe enough to grow', as will be discussed further in Chapter Four.

The concept of 'healing' has been discussed by many contributors. Healing is a practical generalist goal: 'supporting patients in living their lives' (Reeve 2010, 8). It includes facilitating 'relief, repair, and meaning' (Stange, Miller, and McWhinney 2001, 286), rehabilitating the self (Stone 2013b) and 'validating suffering without medicalising misery' (Stone 2013a, 101). Edmund Pellegrino (2006) would open the focus of healing even wider, agreeing with Emperor Claudius's physician (Scribonius Largus) who said the goal of medicine is 'humanitas' (which Pellegrino translates as love and mercy). Trauma researchers make the important distinction between 'getting better and feeling better' (Kluft 2013, 79, Kezelman and Stavropoulos 2019). They point to a more expansive goal than mood or symptom control, or subjective experiences of comfort.

The recovery movement, speaking on behalf of the patient, has defined what processes people report increase their 'recovery'. These processes include hope, healing, empowerment and connection (Jacobson and Greenley 2001); movement from despair to hope, from passive to active sense of self, from others in control to being in personal control, from disconnectedness to connectedness (King, Lloyd, and Meehan 2007); and finding meaning in life, redefining identity and taking responsibility for recovery (Andresen 2000). Interestingly, in view of our focus on the whole person, the origin of the word 'healing' is an Old English word *haelan* which means 'to make whole' (Harper 2020).

Integrative wisdom: Attend to themes

In a clinical encounter, the practitioner needs to keep track of Humpty's needs as well as their own needs for pattern recognition (Launer 1999). This process requires a means to manage attention in the face of complexity. Those who study the clinical method highlight this challenge:

> In the course of the clinical encounter, the clinician attends to some things and ignores others. The clinician's attention is selective and the object of attention is thematic for that moment.
>
> (Sadler and Hulgus 1992, 1316)

If a clinician preserves a focus on a clinical theme or moral goal, or on ethical or pragmatic needs, they can resist their attention being drawn to irrelevant, obvious or fragmented details. Themes connect different disciplines in shared attention across 'different interests, expertise and language' (Carlsen, Von Krogh, and Klev 2004). As well as organising that information coherently and discerning its relative value and importance, attention to themes can help to keep the focus wide, on the breadth of knowledge about the whole person.

An overarching whole person theme directs attention away from 'fragments' such as symptoms or behaviours and towards the whole of Humpty's experience. Choosing a theme that is integral and has proven value to the whole of Humpty's wellbeing will produce useful knowledge relevant across the disciplines. As well as the overarching theme of healing, the concept of *sense of safety* developed in this book is offered to the reader as a transdisciplinary theme relevant to the process, content and priorities of every encounter.

Integrative wisdom: Humble pattern recognition

In the search for what is integral, those caring for Humpty need to be able to see patterns in the interconnections between the parts of the complex whole. This requires attending to the whole and discerning the 'multi-level and non-linear' complexity of each person (McWhinney 1996). It involves attending to sensory, intuitive, experiential and observed information while intentionally avoiding premature diagnostic categorisation or closure (McSherry 1997), or 'the myth of certainty' (Reeve 2010, 8). It also involves 'inductive foraging' – not only looking for pattern recognition but also openly looking for 'pattern failure' (Donner-Banzhoff and Hertwig 2014). It involves 'whole-hearted attending' (Maslow 1954, 195) and 'a kind of modesty about what an individual can and cannot do, knows and does not know' (Pellegrino and Thomasma 1993, 117).

A clear distinction must be made between this form of pattern recognition and categorising. Pattern recognition involves what primary care researchers call 'sense-making' and attending to 'over-arching storylines' (Greenhalgh 2004, 357). It is broad and curious in its scope and tentative in its certainty. In a complex system, it involves a sensory process where reality is probed, sensed and responded to (Kurtz and Snowden 2003). It uses a hermeneutic approach, 'the art of interpretation to create meaning' (McGregor 2018, 191), that looks wide for illumination, before narrowing to define in dynamic cycles of understanding (Ajjawi and Higgs 2007). This is illustrated in Figure 1.2.

Pattern recognition is a part of everyday life. For Humpty, it involves a complex process of appraisal that enables him to make sense of his world, discern his needs, navigate his relationships and decide on his actions. This complex sensory process of appraisal will be discussed in more depth in Chapter Four. Humpty and those caring for him undertake this integrative task daily. This active, sensory and sense-making process is built into the English phrase 'sense of safety'.

Integrative wisdom: Shared language

Speaking the same language as Humpty matters. Technical language can depersonalise and dehumanise care (Todres, Galvin, and Dahlberg 2007). Shared language offers ways to translate meaning between people and across disciplines

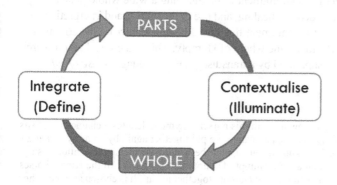

Figure 1.2 Basic hermeneutic circle as per Ajjawi and Higgs (2007).

– 'emergent metaphors of understanding' (Somerville and Rapport 2000, 10). Transdisciplinarity and generalism depend upon and value a shared language (Lynch et al. 2012, Clark 2008). Reeve (2010, 2) describes the shared language when 'practitioners commonly fashion explanations which integrate patient and practitioner conceptual accounts of presented health problems'. Similarly, trans-disciplinary researchers seek a meaningful common language and 'a transcendent language – a meta-language – in which the terms of all the participant disciplines are, or can be, expressed' (Somerville and Rapport 2000, 27).

Ordinary language is a form of metaphor: words used and agreed upon over gen-erations to describe shared embodied experiences in their context. They have been found to 'ring true' as an adequate way to describe and communicate an experience. Humpty, in his native tongue, already uses the phrase 'sense of safety' to describe his appraisal of an integrative whole person experience. In this case, Humpty's language is assumed to be English, but it could just as easily be any other language.

In this book I make a case that the ordinary phrase 'sense of safety' could become a healing goal and clinical theme; it could be the pattern to recognise. It could facilitate 'being with' the person by noticing what Humpty senses and speak-ing in his native tongue. Searching for and building 'sense of safety' could become a shared language for both Humpty and those practitioners who care for him.

The resource of generalist wisdom

Generalist wisdom – to look wide, relate and integrate wisely – could offer the 'huge cultural change' that McWhinney (1996) predicted for healthcare. He saw that the mismatch between the complexity of patients in primary care and the current models of care would alert GPs to the need for change. Generalists highly value the integra-tive craft of holding the subjective experience of both practitioner and patient and attending to breadth of biomedical and psychosocial knowledge (Stange 2009, Henry 2010, Reeve 2010). This is 'the wisdom of a generalist approach that is deeply known but often overlooked in the fragmented world of modern healthcare' (Stange 2009, 198). The concept of *sense of safety* explored in this book is built on this philosophi-cal and practical generalist commitment to maintaining a wide whole person scope through relationships, a focus on healing, and use of integrative and interpretive wis-dom. This is a generalist commitment that could be applied across the community – to transcend the parts, to see the whole of Humpty. This is a clinical and research approach that could be supported by a transdisciplinary language: *sense of safety*.

Notes

1 For those who did not grow up with this nursery rhyme it denotes a character that sits on a wall, falls off into pieces, and cannot be put together again by an army of King's soldiers. Its source is unknown, but it may be a political metaphor. Children sing: 'Humpty Dumpty sat on a wall, Humpty Dumpty had a big fall, All the King's horses and all the King's men, couldn't put Humpty together again'. It is chosen as a metaphor to shift our mindsets, to remember the whole that sometimes gets fragmented.

2 This assumes that Humpty of nursery rhyme fame is male – perhaps an assumption that is not correct!

3 Description of a person who has entered into a voluntary and active therapeutic relationship with a clinician as a citizen with both rights and responsibilities (Marshall 2009); 'persons in context of their own social worlds, listened to, informed, respected, and involved in their care – and their wishes are honored (but not mindfully enacted) during their health care journey' (Epstein and Street 2011, 100).

4 The term 'practitioner' will be used throughout this book to signify all who care for the whole person (rather than addressing only clinicians as the original thesis did).

5 They also mention the goal of seeing the patient through showing interest, sensing feelings, listening to story, touching with sensitivity, and using time wisely (Ventres & Frankel 2015).

6 Although originally a word from the language of the Ngangikurungkurr people of the Daly river area of the Northern Territory of Australia, Professor Judy Atkinson (2002) affirms this is a concept valued across Aboriginal language groups.

References

Ajjawi, Rola, and Joy Higgs. 2007. 'Using hermeneutic phenomenology to investigate how experienced practitioners learn to communicate clinical reasoning'. *The Qualitative Report* 12 (4):612–638.

Allen, J.G. 2013. *Restoring mentalizing in attachment relationships: Treating trauma with plain old therapy*. Washington: American Psychiatric Publishing.

Andresen, Lee W. 2000. 'A useable, trans-disciplinary conception of scholarship'. *Higher Education Research & Development* 19 (2):137–153.

Atkinson, J. 2002. *Trauma trails: Recreating songlines. The transgenerational effects of trauma in indigenous Australia*. Melbourne: Spinifex Press.

Carew, Anna L, and Fern Wickson. 2010. 'The TD wheel: A heuristic to shape, support and evaluate transdisciplinary research'. *Futures* 42 (10):1146–1155.

Carlsen, Arne, George Von Krogh, and Roger Klev. 2004. *Living knowledge: The dynamics of professional service work*. New York: Palgrave Macmillan.

Cassell, E.J. 2010. 'The person in medicine'. *International Journal of Integrated Care* 10 (5):50–52. http://doi.org/10.5334/ijic.489.

Clark, J. 2008. 'The narrative in patient-centred care'. *The British Journal of General Practice: The Journal of the Royal College of General Practitioners* 58 (557):896.

Donner-Banzhoff, Norbert, and Ralph Hertwig. 2014. 'Inductive foraging: Improving the diagnostic yield of primary care consultations'. *The European Journal of General Practice* 20 (1):69–73.

Elwyn, G., A. Lloyd, C. May, T. van der Weijden, A. Stiggelbout, A. Edwards, D.L.T. Frosch, T. Rapley, T. Barr Walsh, S.W. Grande, V. Montori, and R. Epstein 2014. 'Collaborative deliberation: A model for patient care'. *Patient Education and Counselling* 97 (2):158–164. https://doi.org/10.1016/j.pec.2014.07.027.

Epstein, R.M. and R.L. Street. 2011. *The values and value of patient-centered care* 9(2): 100–103.

Epstein, Ronald M. 2014. 'Realizing Engel's biopsychosocial vision: Resilience, compassion, and quality of care'. *The International Journal of Psychiatry in Medicine* 47 (4):275–287.

Epstein, Ronald M., and Anthony L. Back. 2015. 'Responding to suffering'. *JAMA* 314 (24):2623–2624.

Fricker, Miranda. 2007. *Epistemic injustice: Power and the ethics of knowing*. Oxford: Oxford University Press.

Getz, Linn, A.L. Kirkengen, and E. Ulvestad. 2011. 'The human biology-saturated with experience'. *Tidsskr Nor Legeforen* 131 (7):683–687.

Gray, Barbara. 2008. 'Enhancing transdisciplinary research through collaborative leadership'. *American Journal of Preventive Medicine* 35 (2):S124–S132.

Greenhalgh, T. 2004. 'Chapter 20. Meta-narrative mapping: A new approach to the systematic review of complex evidence'. In Brian Hurwitz (ed.), *Narrative research in health and illness*. London: BMJ Publishing.

Harper, D. 2020. 'Heal'. In *Online etymology dictionary*. https://www.etymonline.com/

Henry, Stephen G. 2010. 'Polanyi's tacit knowing and the relevance of epistemology to clinical medicine'. *Journal of Evaluation in Clinical Practice* 16 (2):292–297.

Howie, J.G., David J. Heaney, Margaret Maxwell, and Jeremy J. Walker. 1998. 'A comparison of a patient enablement instrument (PEI) against two established satisfaction scales as an outcome measure of primary care consultations'. *Family Practice* 15 (2):165–171.

Jacobson, N., and D. Greenley. 2001. 'What is recovery? A conceptual model and explication'. *Psychiatric Services (Washington, D.C.)* 52 (4):482–485.

Kezelman, Cathy, and Pam Stavropoulos. 2019. *Practice guidelines for treatment of complex Trauma*. Sydney: Blue Knot Foundation

King, Robert, Chris Lloyd, and Tom Meehan, eds. 2007. *Handbook of psychosocial rehabilitation*. Melbourne: Blackwell Publishing.

Kirkengen, Anna Luise. 2005. 'Encountering particulars: A life in medicine'. *The Permanente Journal* 9 (3):19.

Kluft, Richard P. 2013. Shelter from the *storm*: Processing the Traumatic *memories of* DID/ DDNOS *patients with fractionated abreaction technique*. South Carolina: CreateSpace.

Krieger, Nancy. 2005. 'Embodiment: A conceptual glossary for epidemiology'. *Journal of Epidemiology & Community Health* 59 (5):350–355.

Kurtz, Cynthia F., and David J. Snowden. 2003. 'The new dynamics of strategy: Sense-making in a complex and complicated world'. *IBM Systems Journal* 42 (3):462–483.

Launer, John. 1999. 'Narrative based medicine: A narrative approach to mental health in general practice'. *BMJ: British Medical Journal* 318 (7176):117–119.

Lynch, J.M. 2019. *Sense of safety: A whole person approach to distress*. PhD, Primary Care Clinical Unit, University of Queensland.

Lynch, J.M., D.A. Askew, G.K. Mitchell, and K.L. Hegarty. 2012. 'Beyond symptoms: Defining primary care mental health clinical assessment priorities, content and process'. *Social Science & Medicine* 74 (2):143–149. doi:10.1016/j.socscimed.2011.08.043.

Lynch, J.M., C.F. Dowrick, Pamela Meredith, S.L.T. McGregor, and Mieke Van Driel. 2020. 'Transdisciplinary generalism: Naming the epistemology and philosophy of the generalist'. *Journal of Evaluation in Clinical Practice*, pages 1–10.

Marshall, M. 2009. *Revalidation: a professional imperative. The British Journal of General Practice: the Journal of the Royal College of General Practitioners* 59 (564): 476.

Maslow, A.H. 1954. *Motivation and personality third edition*. Edited by R. Frager, J. Fadiman, C. McReynolds, and R. Cox. New York: Harper Collins Publishers.

McGregor, S.L.T. 2018. 'Philosophical underpinnings of the transdisciplinary research methodology'. *Transdisciplinary Journal of Engineering and Science* 9:182–198.

McIntosh, Thomas Allan, Bonnie Jeffery, and Nazeem Muhajarine. 2010. *Redistributing health: New directions in population health research in Canada*. Vol. 38. Regina, Canada: University of Regina Press.

McSherry, David. 1997. 'Avoiding premature closure in sequential diagnosis'. *Artificial Intelligence in Medicine* 10 (3):269–283.

McWhinney, Ian R. 1996. 'The importance of being different. William Pickles Lecture 1996'. *The British Journal of General Practice* 46 (408):433–436.

Pellegrino, Edmund D. 2006. 'Toward a reconstruction of medical morality'. *The American Journal of Bioethics* 6 (2):65–71.

Pellegrino, Edmund D., and David Thomasma. 1993. *The virtues in medical practice.* New York: Oxford University Press.

Popa, Florin, Mathieu Guillermin, and Tom Dedeurwaerdere. 2015. 'A pragmatist approach to transdisciplinarity in sustainability research: From complex systems theory to reflexive science'. *Futures* 65:45–56.

Reason, Peter, and Hilary Bradbury. 2001. *Handbook of action research: Participative Inquiry and Practice.* London: Sage.

Reeve, J. 2010. 'Interpretive medicine: Supporting generalism in a changing primary care world'. *Occasional Paper Royal College of General Practitioners* 88:1–20.

Reeve, J., T. Blakeman, G.K. Freeman, L.A. Green, P.A. James, P. Lucassen, C.M. Martin, J.P. Sturmberg, and C. van Weel. 2013. 'Generalist solutions to complex problems: Generating practice-based evidence – the example of managing multi-morbidity'. *BMC Family Practice* 14 (1):112. https://doi.org/10.1186/1471-2296-14-112.

Sadler, J.Z., and Y.F. Hulgus. 1992. 'Clinical problem solving and the biopsychosocial model'. *The American Journal of Psychiatry* 149 (10):1315–1323.

Schön, Donald A. 1995. The reflective practitioner: How professionals think in action. Vol. 5126. London: Basic books.

Scott, J.G., D. Cohen, B. DiCicco Bloom, W. Miller, K. Stange, and B. Crabtree 2008. 'Understanding healing relationships in primary care'. *Annals of Family Medicine* 6 (4):315–322.

Somerville, M.A., and D.J. Rapport. 2000. *Transdisciplinarity: Recreating integrated knowledge.* Oxford: Eolss Publishers Co. Ltd.

Stange, Kurt C. 2009. 'The generalist approach'. *The Annals of Family Medicine* 7 (3):198–203.

Stange, Kurt C., William L. Miller, and I. McWhinney. 2001. 'Developing the knowledge base of family practice'. *Family Medicine* 33 (4):286–297.

Stone, Louise. 2013a. 'Making sense of medically unexplained symptoms in general practice: A grounded theory study'. *Mental Health in Family Medicine* 10 (2):101–111.

Stone, Louise. 2013b. 'Reframing chaos: A qualitative study of GPs managing patients with medically unexplained symptoms'. *Australian Family Physician* 42 (7):1–7.

Todres, L., K. Galvin, and K. Dahlberg. 2007. 'Lifeworld-led healthcare: Revisiting a humanising philosophy that integrates emerging trends.' *Medicine, Health Care and Philosophy* 10 (1):53–63.

Ungunmerr, M.R., ed. 1993. *Dadirri: Listening to one another.* Edited by J. Hendricks, and G. Heffernan, *A spirituality of catholic aborigines and the struggle for justice.* Brisbane: Aboriginal and Torres Strait Islander Apostate, Catholic Archdiocese of Brisbane.

Ventres, William B., and Richard M. Frankel. 2015. 'Shared presence in physician-patient communication: A graphic representation'. *Families, Systems, & Health* 33 (3):270–279. http://doi.org/10.1037/fsh0000123.

2 Reductionist barriers to seeing the whole – why can't the King's Men put Humpty together again?

- There are barriers to the King's Men putting Humpty together again
- When Humpty is distressed he cannot sense his 'whole'
- In an attempt to be more certain, practitioners who care for the distressed often narrow their gaze and speak narrowed dialects
- There is a moral imperative to see the whole person

As a general practitioner (GP) or family doctor, I have had the privilege of learning from both biomedical and social science experts. As my interest in the impact of life story on biology grew, I became intrigued as to why good quality science had not been translated into practice – into the real world where I work. Why had the new evidence on the importance of safe relationships for brain function not resulted in changed childcare arrangements? Why had the evidence on the impact of dietary sugar not changed advertising standards? Why had the legitimate theoretical concerns about comorbid psychiatric diagnosis and what some called 'nosologomania' (Ghaemi 2009, 10) not caused a widespread reconceptualisation of the whole field of mental health? Why had the voice of the patient in the recovery literature not shifted health goals? Perhaps those in reductive disciplines had no reason to seek disruption beyond their silo. The UN asserts that:

> Reductive biomedical approaches to treatment that do not adequately address contexts and relationships can no longer be considered compliant with the right to health.
>
> (UN 2017, 17)

Generalism, as discussed in Chapter One, is not reductionist – it looks wide to see the whole person. Generalists have a vested interest in looking across silos of what is known to find patterns to help the whole person in distress toward lifelong wellbeing.

Seeing only a 'part' diminishes the whole

Fifteen years ago (before diabetic educators were the norm), I saw a 45-year-old woman, 'Tanya', for the first time. She had come in to speak about blood results that confirmed her diabetes was out of control, and she would need to start diabetic medication. After a slightly awkward conversation, Tanya left with a prescription. She came six weeks later to confess she was not taking the tablets. Only then did I learn that as a child she had watched her grandmother have multiple amputations as a result of diabetes. Taking a diabetic tablet was an awful symbol. It meant those memories were vivid. These fears overwhelmed her resolve to take the prescription. If only my first contact had looked wider. If only I had looked beyond the blood tests and the diagnosis to what taking diabetic medication symbolised for Tanya and how it linked to her much-loved grandmother. Focusing on the diagnosis and prescription meant I had missed more important information.

Siloed specialised knowledge simultaneously informs and impoverishes understanding of our world. The late Puggy (Arnold) Hunter, an Aboriginal elder, spoke these words that will resonate throughout this book and across cultures:

> There is an urgent need to shift the paradigm of Aboriginal health service delivery away from the current maze of programs and specialists dealing with specific conditions, to a holistic approach that looks at the health of the whole person, the family, and the community.
>
> The 'body parts' approach has been a complete failure in Aboriginal health. There is no use treating the heart or the ears alone, when the whole person is in danger of breaking down ... This means a new way of thinking.
>
> (Hunter 1999, 2)

The 'body parts' approach has dominated modern medicine and influenced our culture. It has influenced how we perceive children's behaviours in schools, workplace wellbeing and health across the community. It has influenced funding, research and the biomedical or sociological solutions we develop. Whole systems and ways of thinking are built around the body parts approach to wellbeing.

Although the body parts approach has many strengths that have improved wellbeing across the globe – from sanitation to hearing aid design – it is clear that it has major limitations. Good quality biomedical research is designed to explore and predict and to be reliable, repeatable and specific. It is objective, reductionist, decontextualised, deterministic and dualist. As outlined in Table 2.1 below, these characteristics, by their nature, exclude other forms of knowledge. Generalist researchers call this the 'blinded medical gaze ... [with its] ... disinterest in subjective experiences' (Kirkengen 2008, 99).

Invisible straightjackets

When people are viewed through a lens of 'body parts' they are diminished. Bravery and stories of adventure, often hidden inside frailty or aggression, are overlooked. Important factors can be missed such as the impacts on life of work,

Table 2.1 Good Quality Biomedicine Values and Excludes (Adapted from Lynch et al. (2020) 'Transdisciplinary Generalism')

Good positivist biomedical research is	It therefore must exclude knowledge about:		Key information lost from whole person assessment
Objective	Subjective inner experience	Perception and meaning	Loss of subjective experience and the voice of the patient/ clinician
Reductionist	Complex patterns processes	Homeostatic regulation	Loss of detailed dynamic attention to the whole person
Decontextualised	Relationships and environment	Other 'confounding variables'	Loss of story, family, community and cultural identity.
Deterministic	Growth	Change dynamics	Loss of humility, agency, meaning-making, spirituality and sense of story over time
Dualist	Integration of mind and body	Organism as a whole	Loss of holism and meaningful connection to the body

finances, family disconnection, conflict with loved ones, vitamin D levels or even loss of a pet. In the words of a GP stakeholder in my PhD research: 'We are leaving out things that people need to get well'. The body parts approach misses the gift of complexity that allows for many small changes across the organism. These small changes can add up to new ways of being in the world that have a profound impact on the wellbeing of a person, their family and the wider community.

Despite being integral to health (Epstein, Quill, and McWhinney 1999), the embodied whole person, their subjective experience and complex relationships with the world are often overlooked by practitioners. Clinicians also describe their own clinical interactions and interpretations as being unaccounted for (and therefore not taught or valued) within this straightjacket that 'incorporates only questions and phenomena that can be controlled, measured, counted and analysed' (Malterud 2001, 397). This ignoring leads to 'narrowly limited clinical realities' (Raskin and Lewandowski 2000, 17) or diagnoses with spurious precision (Wood, Allen, and Pantelis 2009). By their nature, these limitations hinder understanding of the person (Mirowsky and Ross 1989, Hurwitz, Greenhalgh, and Skultans 2004) and increase the risk that psychosocial cues are missed (Salmon et al. 2004), misunderstood, not considered or categorised as 'medically unexplained' (Murray et al. 2016).

As a classification, the phenomenon of 'medically unexplained symptoms' reveals the obvious limitations of the fragmented body parts approach and its consequent inability to see the whole person (Eriksen et al. 2013). Some of the main clinical presentations in general practice involve whole organism dysregulation such as chronic pain, trauma or stress, or indistinct or undifferentiated symptoms, and have either no place, or an awkward place, in the current taxonomy. This diminished and inadequate view of the people we care for is an urgent concern. It matters.

Limited ways of seeing narrow our view of the whole. Prematurely narrowed categorising can make our 'knowing' invalid. Both biomedical and sociological disciplines have made significant improvements to the care of distress, and yet both can constrain holistic knowledge by either 'technical or social reductionism' (Horlick-Jones and Sime 2004, 452). Unless each of these paradigms is aware of their limited scope and learns how to see and value each other, they may constrain breakthroughs in the assessment and treatment of distress.

Maslow (1954, xxx) also warned against these constraints when he wrote that 'truth can be born into an invisible straightjacket'. Some commentators, such as Fricker (2007), go further and frame narrow approaches to the whole person as a 'form of injustice' where knowledge formation (epistemology) and interpretation of evidence (hermeneutics) ignore aspects of the whole. These disciplinary straightjackets are not just of theoretical influence. They impact the conceptualisation of what breadth of understanding is relevant to care of distress, what knowledge is considered reliable, what suffering is considered legitimate and whether collaboration across disciplines is considered valuable or possible.

The King's Men speak different dialects: Can Humpty Dumpty be put back together again?

Approaches to health have become fragmented in an attempt to manage expanding knowledge and pursue certainty and precision. In considering the King's Men – the community charged with care for Humpty's distress – what has happened with the fragmentation of medicine can offer a warning and a way forward for other parts of the community. Humpty is studied and cared for in scattered pieces across different faculties or disciplines and is often spoken about with the use of specialised jargon that separates knowledge from other professions. Of most concern, this process also separates Humpty from an understanding of his own health. Patients often report feeling bewildered and made vulnerable by current theoretically chaotic medical approaches (Stone 2013).

Disciplinary approaches are necessarily reductionist (Horlick-Jones and Sime 2004) with inherent jargon and hierarchies of knowledge value – perhaps made more overt through the evidence-based movement (Mykhalovskiy and Weir 2004). In a bid for respectability, the drive to proceed up the dominant linear hierarchy of evidence has led even those fields devoted to the subjective complexity of the mind to categorise and measure subjective relational processes in a linear classification system. In a multidisciplinary healthcare context that outsources care for the mind to psychiatry and psychology, mental health is consigned to always be a fragment of the whole.

Iona Heath, a GP, points out that disease and unease that do not fit the patterns that reductionist science recognises are often 'invalidated ... belittled and ignored' (1997, 17). Louise Stone names this process 'disease prestige' (2018). When a complex phenomenon is constrained to linear rules of observation, our understanding will be limited. Sue McGregor (2004, 7), a transdisciplinary researcher, reminds us that: 'Simplifying reality to simplify our work is irresponsible'. Within biomedicine this reductionism can lead to wider social issues being 'located within an individual' (mhc). It can influence priorities so that genetic mapping of an individual takes precedence over understanding the health impact of poverty or overcrowding. This reductionist approach to parts of the whole leads to disrespect and language barriers between the King's Men and has an impact on approaches to Humpty's health – those who care for Humpty cannot see him – or even worse, they may claim spuriously to know precisely what they are seeing when all they are seeing is a fragment.

Instead: What if, when anyone saw a distracted child, they could see it was not a disorder in them but in their home? Or, when someone with angina came into the clinic, the clinicians knew it was only a little to do with his cholesterol and a lot to do with his financial stress? What if the whole community could see that suicidality was not about mood but about hope? Or that sadness wasn't a psychiatric diagnosis but grief? Or obesity was due to intergenerational trauma and injustice and not just calories? Or, when someone had repeated neck pain, it wasn't their spine that needed an X-ray but they who needed a new office chair? Or, when someone was jumpy at work, it was nothing to do with their workmates and something to do with their controlling partner? What if, as a community, we committed to addressing and resourcing the whole, rather than focusing on (perhaps the more manageable) parts?

What are the main languages that the King's Men speak?

The disciplines have different ways to value knowledge or what some call 'evidence'. What is researched, noticed and interpreted is influenced by beliefs about reality (ontology), knowledge creation (epistemology), how humans understand what is true (logic) and what is valued (axiology). A fundamental division exists between whether objective (positivist) or subjective (post-positivist) knowledge is considered valuable. This differing set of values influences how knowledge is formed in 'epistemic cultures' (Cetina 2009). Although discussed in more depth elsewhere (Lynch et al. 2020), Table 2.2, 'Ways of "Knowing"', summarises these differences in the languages and values of the King's Men.

Positivism forms knowledge through observation and discovery for the purpose of prediction. It values certainty, linear deductive reasoning and impartiality. It roots what it calls 'evidence' in reductionist processes of excluding what it calls 'variables' (including relationships and context) and in Cartesian (and Greek) separation of the supposedly rational mind from the sensory (and fallible) body and the world it experiences (Barnacle 2001). It sees knowledge derived from the 'disembodied consciousness' (or mind) as more valuable than other forms of knowledge (Barnacle 2001, 5). It reduces the body to an object of study separate

Table 2.2 Ways of 'Knowing'

Ways of 'Knowing'	Positivist	Post-Positivist		Both Positivist and Post-positivist
	Empirical Seeing	Interpretive Listening	Critical Questioning	Transdisciplinary Discerning
Reality (Ontology)	Discoverable Context-free	Conditional Socially constructed	Shaped by politics and power	Multifaceted and in flux
Knowledge (Epistemology)	Observable with the senses Explorable	Co-created Transactional Subjective	Grounded in context and history	Dynamic Emergent Transcendent
Logic (Acceptable Rigour)	Rational Linear Either/Or Explain/Predict	Inductive Understanding	Persuade Emancipate	Inclusive Logic Reconcile contradictions
Values (Axioms)	Objectivity Replicable Reliable	Rich evidence Credible Justifiable Reflexive	Proactive values drive transformation	Integral Interactions Emergence Hidden Third

(adapted from Lynch et al. (2020) 'Transdisciplinary Generalism')

from the mind. Michel Foucault (1967, 188) called this 'experience reduced to silence by positivism'. It is amenable to measurement and understanding causality and has contributed to significant improvements across society. It underpins biotechnical conceptions of health and strict hierarchies of valid knowledge or 'evidence'. This form of knowledge is valued and offers gifts to the community from the boardroom to the school room or hospital.

Post-positivist knowledge, on the other hand, values complex understandings of relationships and context for the purpose of interpretation. It values knowledge formed (or constructed) between people and attends to meaning, senses, experience and subjective perceptions. It uses inductive reasoning and understands that all knowledge is imperfect. It acknowledges the bias and influence of all those who contribute to forming knowledge (there are no observers, only participants in this approach to knowledge). This form of knowledge is often used in psychosocial research. It values subjectivity and complexity and is suspicious of processes that privilege reason over experience. The post-positivist social sciences do, however, have the potential for 'sociological imperialism' (Strong 1979) when they view their perspective as the whole rather than as part of the whole.

As a clinician trained in biomedicine, I am aware of disrespect from both sides of the biomedicine and social science 'fragments' – the social sciences are often dismissed as 'soft' science ('complex' may be more accurate) by those who proffer 'hard' science, by which they mean 'real' science ('linear' may be more descriptive). Biomedicine is discussed among social scientists in shared assumptions of the inadequacy of the 'medical model'. These fields of research and practice rarely acknowledge the validity of the other as part of the whole (even when placed next to one another in mixed-methods research). While both have valuable theoretical contributions to the philosophy of generalism, and their integration is part of the experiential skill set of the generalist (often taught through a hidden curriculum by their patients), they are yet to be integrated into coherent primary care approaches to the whole.

Cassell's understanding of the person assumes an integration of both positivist biomedical knowledge and post-positivist psychosocial knowledge. Generalist practitioners need to be able to accommodate and attune to relational, contextual and subjective information at the same time as valuing objective, decontextualised, biomedical (or other factual) knowledge (Reeve 2010). The key areas that need to be included in research or care for the whole person are included in the *whole person knowledge map* in Figure 2.1. Positivist (outer concepts) and post-positivist (inner concepts) are depicted as part of the knowing required to offer whole person care. This approach is not anti-biomedical or anti-social science. Instead, it honours the skills of those who integrate both approaches and discern the breadth and depth of what is most important. All these aspects of Humpty are important, whether in the classroom, policy planning, the healthcare clinic, the research department or the boardroom. This map will define the scope of an adequate whole person approach to distress and wellbeing, as developed in this book.

This whole person awareness enables 'diagnosis' – built on Greek words that mean comprehensive or thorough (*Dia*) and knowledge (*Gnosis*) – not the more

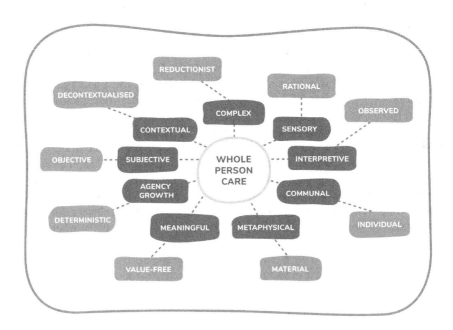

Figure 2.1 Whole person knowledge map.

limiting 'diagnosis of disease' (Sturmberg and Martin 2007, xi, Harding, Wait, and Scrutton 2015, 1). This is the privilege of the practitioner on the border of biomedicine and community: the skill of considering the whole – of recognising and bearing witness to 'the poetry of life in the science of the ordinary' (Stange, Miller, and McWhinney 2001, 286), despite practical limitations (Cape et al. 2008). This skill is relevant for all practitioners who seek to care for the whole person.

Predicted innovation sparked by generalism

Ian McWhinney expected that innovation would come as the fault line between the mind and body of reductionist biomedical or body parts approaches was tested by generalists in the real-life complexity of their community. He described generalists as:

> prisoners of an unreformed clinical method and the language of linear causation and mind/body dualism. The fault line that runs through the affect-denying clinical method which dominates the modern medical school.
>
> (McWhinney 1996, 436)

Reforming this clinical method and our communal attitude to the whole person will require getting the disciplinary giants to dance (Carlsen, Von Krogh, and Klev 2004). It will require transdisciplinary and generalist philosophy and skills to understand the different dialects of the King's Men (the disciplinary giants) and invite them onto the dance floor of shared understanding and the shared language of *sense of safety* (Reeve 2010, Lynch et al. 2012, Goldberg 1992, Kirkengen et al. 2014).

References

Barnacle, Robyn. 2001. 'Phenomenology and wonder.' In *Phenomenology*, edited by R. Barnacle. Vol 3. Melbourne: RMIT Publishing.

Cape, J., E. Morris, M. Burd, and M. Buszewicz. 2008. 'Complexity of GPs' explanations about mental health problems: Development, reliability, and validity of a measure.' *The British Journal of General Practice* 58 (551):403–410.

Carlsen, Arne, George Von Krogh, and Roger Klev. 2004. *Living knowledge: The dynamics of professional service work*. New York: Palgrave Macmillan.

Cetina, Karin Knorr. 2009. *Epistemic cultures: How the sciences make knowledge*. Cambridge, MA: Harvard University Press.

Epstein, Ronald M., Timothy E. Quill, and Ian R. McWhinney. 1999. 'Somatization reconsidered: Incorporating the patient's experience of illness.' *Archives of Internal Medicine* 159 (3):215–222.

Eriksen, Thor Eirik, Roger Kerry, Stephen Mumford, Svein Anders Noer Lie and Rani Lill Anjum. 2013. 'At the borders of medical reasoning: Aetiological and ontological challenges of medically unexplained symptoms.' *Philosophy, Ethics, and Humanities in Medicine* 8 (1):11. https://doi.org/10.1186/1747-5341-8-11.

Foucault. 1967. *Madness and civilisation*. London: Routledge.

Fricker, Miranda. 2007. *Epistemic injustice: Power and the ethics of knowing*. Oxford: Oxford University Press.

Ghaemi, S.N. 2009. 'Nosologomania: DSM & Karl Jaspers' critique of Kraepelin.' *Philosophy, Ethics, and Humanities in Medicine* 4 (1):10. https://doi.org/10.1186/1747 -5341-4-10.

Goldberg, David. 1992. 'A classification of psychological distress for use in primary care settings.' *Social Science & Medicine* 35 (2):189–193.

Harding, Ed, Suzanne Wait, and Jonathan Scrutton. 2015. *The state of play in person-centred care*. London: The Health Policy Partnership.

Heath, I., ed. 1997. *The mystery of general practice*. London: Nuffield Provincial Hospital Trust.

Horlick-Jones, Tom, and Jonathan Sime. 2004. 'Living on the border: Knowledge, risk and transdisciplinarity.' *Futures* 36 (4):441–456.

Hunter, Puggy (Arnold). 1999. 'Searching for a new way of thinking in aboriginal health.' *NACCHO News* 3 (July):1–2.

Hurwitz, B., T. Greenhalgh, and V. Skultans, eds. 2004. *Narrative research in health and illness*. Melbourne: Blackwell Publishing.

Kirkengen, Anna Luise. 2008. 'Inscriptions of violence: Societal and medical neglect of child abuse – impact on life and health.' *Medicine, Health Care and Philosophy* 11 (1):99–110.

Kirkengen, Anna Luise, Bente Prytz Mjolstad, Linn Getz, Elling Ulvestad, and Irene Hetlevik. 2014. 'Can person-free medical knowledge inform person-centered medical practice.' *European Journal for Person Centered Healthcare* 2:32–36.

Lynch, J.M., D.A. Askew, G.K. Mitchell, and K.L. Hegarty. 2012. 'Beyond symptoms: Defining primary care mental health clinical assessment priorities, content and process.' *Social Science & Medicine* 74 (2):143–9. doi:10.1016/j.socscimed.2011.08.043.

Lynch, J.M., C.F. Dowrick, Pamela Meredith, S.L.T. McGregor, and Mieke Van Driel. 2020. 'Transdisciplinary generalism: Naming the epistemology and philosophy of the generalist.' *Journal of Evaluation in Clinical Practice*: 1–10. doi: 10.1111/jep.13446.

Malterud, Kirsti. 2001. 'The art and science of clinical knowledge: Evidence beyond measures and numbers.' *The Lancet* 358 (9279):397–400.

Maslow, A.H. 1954. *Motivation and personality third edition*. Edited by R. Frager, J. Fadiman, C. McReynolds, and R. Cox. New York: Harper Collins Publishers.

McGregor, S.L.T. 2004. 'The nature of transdisciplinary research and practice.' In *Kappa Omicron Nu human sciences working paper series*. Halifax: Mount Saint Vincent University.

McWhinney, Ian R. 1996. 'The importance of being different. William Pickles Lecture 1996.' *The British Journal of General Practice* 46 (408):433–436.

Mirowsky, John, and Catherine E. Ross. 1989. 'Psychiatric diagnosis as reified measurement.' *Journal of Health and Social Behavior* 30 (1):11–25.

Murray, Alexandra M., Anne Toussaint, Astrid Althaus, and Bernd Löwe. 2016. 'The challenge of diagnosing non-specific, functional, and somatoform disorders: A systematic review of barriers to diagnosis in primary care.' *Journal of Psychosomatic Research* 80:1–10.

Mykhalovskiy, Eric, and Lorna Weir. 2004. 'The problem of evidence-based medicine: Directions for social science.' *Social Science & Medicine* 59 (5):1059–1069.

Raskin, Jonathan D., and Adam M. Lewandowski. 2000. 'The construction of disorder as human enterprise.' In *Constructions of disorder*, edited by Robert A. Neimeyer. Washington, DC: American Psychological Association.

Reeve, J. 2010. 'Interpretive medicine: Supporting generalism in a changing primary care world.' *Occasional Paper Royal College of General Practitioners* 88:1–20.

Salmon, P., C.F. Dowrick, A. Ring, and G.M. Humphris. 2004. 'Voiced but unheard agendas: Qualitative analysis of the psychosocial cues that patients with unexplained symptoms present to general practitioners.' *The British Journal of General Practice* 54 (500):171–176.

Stange, Kurt C., William L. Miller, and I. McWhinney. 2001. 'Developing the knowledge base of family practice.' *Family Medicine* 33 (4):286–297.

Stone, Louise. 2013. 'Reframing chaos: A qualitative study of GPs managing patients with medically unexplained symptoms.' *Australian Family Physician* 42 (7):1–7.

Stone, Louise. 2018. 'Disease prestige and the hierarchy of suffering.' *Medical Journal of Australia* 208 (2):60–62.

Strong, Phil M. 1979. 'Sociological imperialism and the profession of medicine a critical examination of the thesis of medical imperialism.' *Social Science & Medicine. Part A: Medical Psychology & Medical Sociology* 13:199–215.

Sturmberg, Joachim P., and Carmel M. Martin. 2007. *The foundations of primary care: Daring to be different.* Oxford; Seattle: Radcliffe.

UN. 2017. *Report of the Special Rapporteur on the right of everyone to the enjoyment of the highest attainable standard of physical and mental health.* Edited by Human Rights Council. UN General Assembly.

Wood, Stephen J., Nicholas B. Allen, and Christos Pantelis. 2009. *The neuropsychology of mental illness.* New York: Cambridge University Press.

3 Transcending disciplinary silos

The new science is leading us to see all of Humpty at once

- Seeing Humpty all at once requires a shared language and coherent philosophical approaches to the whole
- Neither biopsychosocial nor transdiagnostic approaches are philosophically coherent enough to see the whole of Humpty
- Transdisciplinary approaches include many islands of knowledge culture transcending disciplinary cultures for the sake of seeing the whole of Humpty

As we discovered with the King's Men in Chapter Two, there are distinct language dialects and knowledge cultures among the disciplines. These different cultures and languages remind me of the Indonesian archipelago where I spent my high school years. This archipelago is made up of thousands of islands with many local languages and cultures. When Indonesia became a nation-state, the central government promoted the use of a trade language called Bahasa Indonesia. This language was simple and easy to learn. It was taught in schools and used in the marketplace. It allowed people from different language groups to communicate using the shared trade language, while allowing each island to keep its own language. It encouraged national unity and shared identity.

Unlike Indonesia's many islands, Humpty is already a unity. He is an interconnected whole. He has an ancient interconnecting language – he communicates with himself through metabolic, sensory and hormonal feedback loops. As we will discuss later, he already uses a native language around the universal experience of threat: 'sense of safety'. This way of making sense of his whole-of-person experiences could become a kind of trade language for those who seek to care for the wellbeing of the whole of Humpty. Unfortunately, it is the detailed and specific ways that we have studied Humpty, often removed from his natural relational environment, that have led to different islands of knowledge and jargon that are now often used routinely to describe him. Sometimes they claim to have superior evidence about who Humpty is, or even claim that it is the complete story – not even acknowledging the existence of the other islands. These fragmented dialects are an artefact; they do not facilitate an accurate view of Humpty. As Kirkengen et al. (2016, 500) declares:

Medical thinking needs to be changed, not by bridging the gap between human subjectivity and materiality, but by realising that these two were never separate.

(Kirkengen et al. 2016, 500)

Some would argue that crossing the disciplinary culture barriers, to search for metanarratives or theoretical integration of parts, is not possible or is a foolish attempt to see an elusive whole (Lyotard 1984). Others remind us that 'human experiences, and thus more generally human nature, are stable enough to make at least some provisional generalisations about them' (Low 2010, 199). Transdisciplinary researchers remind us 'it is as dangerous to venture into alien disciplines as it is not to' (Hamberger 2004, 488). In this chapter we will consider principles about how knowledge is managed that offer a way forward – away from fragmentation – towards a shared language.

Why the biopsychosocial model is not enough

At present the biopsychosocial model is the main theoretical framework used to teach the organisation of knowledge about the whole person in medical training. George Engel proposed the idea of a biopsychosocial model as a response to what he called a medical crisis – responding to those who urged the removal of the 'psychosociological underbrush' from medicine's quest to deal with '"real" diseases' (Engel 1977, 129). He was aware biomedical dogma may resist change, so he drew links to general systems theory as a solution to biology's molecular reductionism.

Although designed to bridge the gap between biology and psychosocial ways of knowing, the biopsychosocial model has been critiqued for the way it does not attend to how to integrate different knowledge cultures (Ghaemi 2007) or attend to life story and subjective experience (Brendel 2007). Using the metaphor of the Indonesian islands, the biopsychosocial model makes no attempt to use a shared trade language. Instead, it in effect brings the dialects or cultures from a few different islands together without any translator present. Even more concerning, the dominant biomedical approach to knowledge is often used to make sense of this untranslated information.

In practice the biopsychosocial model also just brings one or two representatives from the hundreds of knowledge islands that represent 'psycho' or 'social' knowledge and interprets them as though they represent the whole group. Some name this limitation of the biopsychosocial model 'reifying' – making something complex and abstract into something concrete and named and supposedly simple (like the word 'social'). In this way it is still very reductionist – it narrows the breadth of insight of complex knowledge cultures to a few simple untranslated phrases. It then makes the awful assumption that it has represented or understood the whole – that the terms bio, psycho and social are comprehensive and unitary (Waterman 2014).

Although it is acknowledged that the biopsychosocial model has 'broaden[ed] the scope of the physician's gaze' (Reeve et al. 2013, 8), it can only partially address the 'dominant biomedical notions that (implicitly or explicitly) define the human body as a biological object devoid of history or experience' (Kirkengen and Thornquist 2012, 1095). This may explain why the biopsychosocial approach has been called an 'empty catchword with little methodological bite' (Sadler and Hulgus 1992, 1315) and simply 'rhetoric' (Dowrick et al. 1996, 105). It may also explain why despite the biopsychosocial model's 'status as "part of the ideology of medicine" it is little used by clinicians' (Waterman 2014, 211). Ghaemi (2009, 3) suggests:

> The biopsychosocial model is seen as an antidote, yet it might equally be a cause, failing to provide convincing conceptual or empirical grounds to resist the biologisation of psychiatry. The problem exists, perhaps, in a failure of the model itself, not a failure to implement it, as many presume.

One of the stakeholders in my doctoral research described the biopsychosocial model as 'tokenism' (gp) and the biomedical model as a 'very old fashioned way of thinking' (gp). He was intuitively aware of the theoretical inadequacies of the biopsychosocial model as he reflected on his generalist clinical practice.

Why transdiagnostic approaches are not enough

Within the 'body part' of mental health, there has been a growing unease with the old-fashioned traditional psychiatric classification systems that rely on positivist approaches to evidence. There is a shift away from disease classification frameworks towards new neurobiological frameworks, transdiagnostic approaches and diagnoses that acknowledge life story or biology. These approaches appear more holistic as they refer to domains, spectra, the human connectome and transdiagnostic processes.

Transdiagnostic approaches, however, are intradisciplinary; they do not transcend disciplinary knowledge barriers and therefore do not include the whole person. If we reflect on the trade language metaphor, these approaches seem to be finding patterns across a few islands while continuing to ignore other islands – almost like a sub-tribe that does not consider the rest of the nation. Transdiagnostic processes within 'mental health' do not address concerns that psychiatric diagnoses are 'so far removed from biological reality', are 'arbitrary' (Kotov et al. 2017, 457) and offer such a 'poor fit to the latent structure of psychopathology' (Buckholtz and Meyer-Lindenberg 2012, 993) that they 'impede clinically useful scientific discovery'(Buckholtz and Meyer-Lindenberg 2012, 993). They also continue to reify the term 'mental' as though there is such a thing: a mind separated from context, physiology, relationship and meaning.

Transdiagnostic insights may be helpful – as we will examine later in this chapter – but they are not enough to offer a view of the whole person. They only consider a part of Humpty and they do not offer a coherent approach to how to consider relationships, meaning and context alongside subjective experience or neurobiology. Transdiagnostic approaches also do not address the fundamental philosophical issue of how to include diverse epistemic (or knowledge) cultures in order to see the whole.

Shift in research and practice: A paradigm changing

There is a shift within healthcare, education and business away from old-fashioned positivist biomedical or even biopsychosocial ways of thinking towards acknowledging the subjective experience or culture of the observer or practitioner. This is a philosophical shift towards post-positivist approaches.

Clinically, post-positivist approaches attend to patient voice and agency, increasing awareness of the person in the clinical encounter. These approaches include consumer consultation and person-centred, relationship-centred, goal-oriented and strengths-based care (Blundo 2001, Reuben and Tinetti 2012, Mezzich, Salloum, et al. 2010, Dewar and Nolan 2013, Reeve 2018, Mezzich, Snaedal, et al. 2010, Donner-Banzhoff 2018). Attitudes such as cultural humility and respect for other disciplines in multidisciplinary teams and interprofessional learning are also informed by this post-positivist approach to knowledge. Approaches to the patient and the clinical method, such as 'narrative medicine' (Charon 2006) and 'interpretive medicine' (Reeve 2010), are built on post-positivist philosophies. They offer a widening view of Humpty, yet they also exclude knowledge islands – the physicality of positivist biomedical cultures. Similar to positivist ignoring of the personhood and experience of the clinician as assumed impartial observer, post-positivist approaches often also exclude the voice and experience (and culture) of the practitioner in their drive to be patient-centred. These post-positivist approaches still do not attempt to integrate positivist and post-positivist knowledge cultures.

Coherent approaches to the whole:
Including knowledge cultures

Of course, there are limitations to how much anyone, even Humpty himself, can 'see' or 'know' the whole. This is one of the tensions and inherent uncertainties of less reductionist ways of seeing. There are therefore philosophical considerations when you seek to transcend knowledge cultures in order to attend to the whole person. This requires not only including both positivist and post-positivist knowledge but also offering philosophically coherent ways to discern how to do this complex interpretive and integrative task. As discussed below, clinical pragmatism, critical realism, indigenous philosophy, hermeneutic phenomenology and transdisciplinarity offer approaches that align with generalist philosophy and point towards seeing the whole.

Clinical pragmatism is a legitimate research methodology that supports the philosophical validity and principles of generalist ways of knowing, linking positivist and post-positivist knowledge. Clinical pragmatism highly values *pragmatic* outcomes, *plural* sources of information, *participatory* process and *provisional* conclusions. A generalist practitioner would easily be able to see these principles and processes in everyday practice. Clinical pragmatism focuses on pragmatic outcomes, focusing on results rather than commitment to any particular theory. This aligns with pragmatic generalist therapeutic goals that include building 'a sense of integrity and wholeness' (Hutchinson 2011, 1), 'general level of personal integration' (Enns et al. 1998, 247) and 'enabl[ing] patients to engage or re-engage with their lives as social beings' (Dowrick 2009, 1146).

Like generalism, clinical pragmatism defines its validity through the breadth of awareness: it gathers *plural* sources of information in order to include explanatory concepts from different knowledge cultures. Clinical pragmatism includes the influence of both Humpty and the practitioner in the *participatory* process of understanding and interpreting knowledge. Similarly, generalist wariness of premature categorisation aligns with *provisional* attitudes to knowledge, remaining open to new information (Lewis 2006, Brendel 2007, Lewis 2014). These principles are ways to protect against the limitations of biological or sociological reductionism, including the biopsychosocial model or transdiagnostic processes.

Critical realism also offers another philosophical approach to the whole. It maintains a provisional attitude to knowledge and acknowledges the limitations and bias of the observer. It also critiques positivism for ignoring social influences while critiquing post-positivism for over-acknowledging social influences (Archer et al. 2013). Reeve (2010) has made a case for the closely aligned philosophy of subtle realism (Maxwell 2002) as a philosophically robust way for generalists to determine value amongst diverse forms of knowledge. In her interpretive medicine approach to knowledge, she identified the importance of robust descriptive, interpretive, theoretical, generalisable and evaluative knowing (Reeve 2010).

Indigenous ways of knowing have the benefit of a long history of seeing Humpty as a whole, embedded in his community and country. Philosophically, these approaches attend to interconnections between mind and body, family and culture, country and spirit. The Indigenous Australian Social Emotional Wellbeing (SEWB) framework describes this way of knowing (Gee et al. 2014). In this model, self is valued as 'inseparable from, and embedded within, family and community' (Gee et al. 2014, 57). This model also includes an understanding of social, political and historical determinants of health.

Phenomenology is a robust philosophical tradition beyond the scope of this book. I will mention *hermeneutic phenomenology* as it describes ways of understanding the complex task of staying open to new information that are part of the skillset of the generalist. This approach, as mentioned in Chapter One, looks wide to the whole for illumination and then narrows to define a part in a constant cycle of searching for patterns or phenomena (Ajjawi and Higgs 2007). A practitioner ascribing to these approaches is committed to being open and willing to be disproven by new information (Augsburg 2014, Barnacle 2001). This approach also highly values wonder, genuine engagement, collaboration, 'responsiveness'

(Barnacle 2001, 22) and the search for rich common meanings (Barnacle 2001, 24) – knowing *with* Humpty.

Hermeneutic phenomenology has similarities to the process of generalist knowing: looking wide, tuning in sensitively to small changes to enable early detection and intervention while at the same time narrowing for pragmatic decision-making. McWhinney calls this 'clinical expertise of the highest order' (McWhinney 1964, ix) that cannot be learned in specialist settings. This capacity to notice widely, to hold knowledge as provisional and to reflect on what is missing is a key element of transdisciplinary and generalist approaches to the whole.

Transcending disciplinary silos: Where the new science is leading us

When I tell clinicians and academics that there is a new transdisciplinary field of study called psychoneuroimmunoendocrinology (PNIE), they often laugh. Those working inside silos are unaware of the careful scientific work of those who cross disciplinary cultural barriers to reveal patterns of interconnection. The transdisciplinary field of psychoneuroimmunology offers ways forward in key areas of health that do not have answers. This way of seeing could help the practitioner and researcher as they attempt to understand pressing concerns such as indigenous life expectancy influenced by transgenerational trauma; asthma, eczema or inflammatory bowel disease affected by life stressors; work productivity affected by management processes; or multimorbidity clustering in the socially disadvantaged (Schiøtz et al. 2017). This lack of awareness of a potentially useful and robust body of research is just more evidence of how we are locked into disciplines. The task of seeing the whole is made much more difficult when Humpty is already prepackaged in fragments in the ways that we research and encounter him.

As mentioned in Chapter One, my doctoral research drew direct correlations between generalism and transdisciplinarity (Lynch et al. 2020, Lynch 2019). Transdisciplinary research highly values shared language, participatory process and the development of real-world outcomes (McGregor, 2004, 2015, 2018). Adding to the earlier definition of transdisciplinarity, it can be understood as:

> scientific enquiry that cuts 'across disciplines', integrating and synthesizing content, theory and methodology from any discipline which will shed light on the research questions ... developing methodologies that can be used to reintegrate knowledge ... to enable different questions to be asked.
>
> (Gray 2008, S124)

Transdisciplinarity is not the dismissal of disciplinary knowledge; instead, it is a process of reconciliation and dialogue, inviting solutions to complex problems beyond disciplinary boundaries (Nicolescu, Morin, and de Freitas 1994). Using the trade language metaphor, transdisciplinarity seeks to provide a language that can enfranchise every island culture a welcome part of the national whole. It sees anything less than this as incomplete. This is a key philosophical position of anyone seeking to care for the whole person.

There are two schools of transdisciplinarity: the practical Zurich school that uses co-creation and community consultation to transcend traditional academic disciplines, and the philosophical or theoretical Nicolescuian school. This philosophical school, as outlined in Table 2.2 in Chapter Two and expanded in Table 3.1, does not simply acknowledge positivist and post-positivist knowledge. It approaches both with a coherent logic, epistemology, ontology and axiology. It includes forms of knowledge that highly value discernment (as well as the seeing, listening and questioning of the other paradigms). It includes forms of knowledge that are often disregarded – such as spiritual, artistic, indigenous and other non-academic ways of meaning-making. It includes intuitive, sensory, experiential and lived forms of knowledge that are shared by patient, clinician and other significant stakeholders (Klein 2015, Christie 2006, Baxi 2000, Polk 2014, Lynch et al. 2020). Transdisciplinarity values inclusive logic (not Aristotelian either/or logic), remains aware of 'Multiple Levels of Reality', and uses what it calls the 'Hidden Third' to unify, transcend and reconcile different ways of knowing.

Table 3.1 Transdisciplinary Philosophy
   (Adapted from Lynch et al. (2020) 'Transdisciplinary Generalism')

Ways of 'Knowing'	**Both Positivist (seeing) AND Post-positivist (listening and questioning)**
	Transdisciplinary
	Discerning
Reality (Ontology)	**Multiple Levels of Reality**
	Multifaceted and in flux
	Potential rich **Hidden Third**
	Mediation of Subjective and Objective information
	Contradictions can be temporarily reconciled[1]
Knowledge	Knowledge as **Emergent Complexity**[2]
(Epistemology)	Dynamic, in flux, moving, and changing
	Emergent, co-created, iterative
	Knowledge is Complex and Embodied[3]
	Knowledge is transcendent as those involved create space for new ideas to emerge[3]
Logic	Inclusive Logic
(Acceptable Rigour)	Logic of the **Included Middle**
	Both/and replaces Aristotelian either /or logic of exclusion
	Reconcile contradictions through unexpected but welcomed integration of facts and perspectives[4]
Values	Integral
(Axioms)	Interactions
	Emergence[5]
	Interactive Hidden Third[4]

[1]McGregor 2015, 2018, 2017.
[2]Nicolescu and Ertas 2013.
[3]McGregor 2015.
[4]McGregor 2018.
[5]McGregor 2011.

These theoretical concepts offer some understanding of the sophistication of generalist approaches to knowledge. Like generalism, transdisciplinarity seeks to understand what is integral (Lynch et al. 2020).

Transdisciplinary inquiry has had increasing influence in addressing complex communal problems (Bernstein 2015). There is a growing application to healthcare (Gibbs 2015), including by those suggesting transdisciplinarity as an 'intellectual foundation' for generalist research (Martin 2003, 905) and a 'scientific essential' to counter specialised knowledge fragmentation (Hamberger 2004, 487). Carmel Martin sees links between transdisciplinarity and generalism as they are both 'open, participatory, respectful and focussed on the real world' (Martin 2003, 905).

Transdisciplinary philosophy validates generalist philosophy and answers calls from primary care clinicians to define their own complex whole person approach (Reeve 2010, Lynch et al. 2012, Goldberg 1992, Kirkengen et al. 2014). Generalists seek congruent frameworks (Johansen and Risor 2017, Reeve et al. 2013) that acknowledge that separation of objective and subjective knowledge is an artefact of scientism[1] – they were 'never separate' (Kirkengen et al. 2016, 500). They call for 'refining and applying transdisciplinary, multimethod, participatory research approaches to answering important questions' (Stange, Miller, and McWhinney 2001, 294). There is a need to transgress disciplines to look beyond the presenting complaint (as GPs frame it) (Thomas, Best, and Mitchell 2020), or the known disciplinary knowledge, to 'reality that is beneath and beyond the subject's experience' (Barnacle 2001, 19).

Identifying phenomena that impact the whole

Even though in many cases it is not built on transdisciplinary philosophical approaches to the whole, there is a growing body of research that transgresses traditional boundaries. Some of these areas of research have clear biomedical or sociological roots, while others are insights from other generalist traditions or emerge from the study of processes that cannot be confined to one discipline or knowledge culture (e.g., multimorbidity or trauma). Many of these insights do not acknowledge the different knowledge cultures that they are attempting to integrate, or, as is the case with transdiagnostic approaches, they do not acknowledge that they are only part of a wider whole. They do, however, offer knowledge that points to a wide whole. This final section of the chapter is a short collation of insights into the whole person that have contributed to the ideas presented in later chapters. These insights represent the beginnings of shared language among the islands of knowledge culture.

Internationally, in research and practice, there is a shift towards more embodied (Kirkengen and Thornquist 2012), sensory (Ogden, Minton, and Pain 2006), neurobiological (Schore 1996, Porges 2011, Cuthbert and Insel 2013), relational (Haggerty, Hilsenroth and Vala-Stewart 2009, Bowlby 1977) and sense-making (Neimeyer 2001) ways of understanding the person. New effective sensorimotor (Fisher 2011), attachment (Cassidy and Shaver 1999), trauma specific (Courtois and Ford 2014), emotion-focused (Butler and Randall 2013) and meaning-making (Park 2010) treatments are also widening understanding and treatment options by seeing more of Humpty's whole.

There is growing scientific understanding of the complex link between biomedical processes and psychosocial experiences (both past and present) (Kirkengen and Thornquist 2012). These include the research into the phenomena of stress (McEwen 2007), trauma (Felitti et al. 1998, Kirkengen 2010), loss (Casey, Dowrick, and Wilkinson 2001), interpersonal violence, medically unexplained symptoms, chronic pain, somatisation, social determinants of health, adverse childhood experiences, multimorbidity, allostatic load, human rights or social justice or equity informed care (Browne et al. 2012), amongst others. This research is revealing a direct link between life experience and health (Anda et al. 2006) – including longevity (Felitti et al. 1998). It is also spawning new fields of research that often reflect their approach to the whole – for example, psychophysiology emerging from the more biological stress research and interpersonal neurobiology emerging from the more relational attachment literature.

The clinical and research areas of coping systems (Moos 1984, Skinner and Zimmer-Gembeck 2007), adaptation (Windle and Woods 2004), salutogenesis (Antonovsky 1987) and resilience (Moser et al. 2019, Cosco, Howse and Brayne 2017) also add transdisciplinary understanding. These ways of seeing the whole person's capacity to adapt can offer a transformational rather than deterministic approach to diagnostic processes.

Research in the field of multimorbidity (Harris, Dennis, and Pillay 2013, Sturmberg et al. 2017) also considers many aspects of the whole person. Multimorbidity is the same theoretical inconsistency to biomedicine as comorbidity is to psychiatry – revealing nosological or diagnostic incoherence. Research in this area seeks to understand patterns that have previously been ignored, leading to more holistic ways of seeing the person. Discipline-bound practical (pragmatic) frameworks from generalist traditions such as those grounded in occupational therapy (Hagedorn 1992), nursing (Wing et al. 1998), palliative care (Anandarajah 2008) or social work (Healy 2014) also help the clinician to see the whole person.

New phenomena identified in the 'body part' of mental health

Shifts in conceptualisation of the mind and its interaction with the whole are an essential substrate for paradigm change. Although not addressing the whole person, these insights from a few knowledge islands are relevant to the whole and are therefore considered here.

The new dimensional and neurobiological Research Domains Criteria (RDoC), developed through the National Institute for Mental Health (NIMH) in the United States (Cuthbert and Insel 2013), replace the psychiatric Diagnostic Statistical Manual (DSM) for research purposes. They include consideration of 'sensori-motor, cognitive, arousal and regulation, negative and positive valence systems, and social processes' (NIMH 2020). Importantly for our later discussion of distress, they clearly outline an acknowledgement of the impact of threat on human behaviour and functioning and acknowledge that threat can be evoked from either internal subjective or external stimuli. Their 'negative valence' domain includes acute threat (fear); potential threat (anxiety); sustained threat; loss; and frustrative nonreward. The RDoC has been critiqued for lack of clinical applicability (Kotov et al. 2017) but has the potential to contribute to an understanding of *sense of safety*, as will be referenced in later chapters.

The field referred to by some as 'transdisciplinary psychiatry' (McGorry et al. 2018), or 'quantitative psychiatric nosology' (Kotov et al. 2017, 458) or the Hierarchical Taxonomy of Psychopathology (HiTOP) does attend to internalising (negative affectivity), thought disorder (psychoticism), disinhibited externalising, antagonistic externalising, detachment and somatoform spectra (Kotov et al. 2017, Krueger and Eaton 2015, 29). This field is still wedded to psychiatric diagnostic frameworks and is missing awareness of context, story and subjective embodied experience but can offer insights into what Humpty is experiencing.

Neurobiologists are also turning away from traditional reductionist psychiatric classification and attending to the 'human connectome' in an attempt to 'synthesise available genetic, neuroimaging and clinical data' (Buckholtz and Meyer-Lindenberg 2012, 999). Although positivist and without a clear way to integrate that information with an understanding of the whole of Humpty, they do identify neural networks involved in social functioning, motivation, cognition and affect.

There is research into both the mechanisms and descriptions of a range of 'psychological transdiagnostic phenomena' (Sauer-Zavala et al. 2017, 129) and new processes to examine them (Forgeard et al. 2011). Examples of these transdiagnostic processes mentioned in the literature are noted in Table 3.2.

There is an increased diagnostic awareness of life story, even in psychiatric diagnostic categories. The DSM diagnostic categories of Dissociation, Post Traumatic Stress Disorder, Borderline Personality Disorder and the proposed Developmental Trauma Disorder acknowledge the traumatic aetiology of the psychopathology (Kate and Dorahy 2019). Although the new ICD-11 diagnosis of Complex Post Traumatic Stress Disorder (C-PTSD) still does not acknowledge subjective forms of stress, it at least acknowledges the impact of adverse events on emotion regulation, sense of self and interpersonal relationships (Maercker et al. 2013). Trauma researchers have consistently identified a person's stressful life story as a common thread that may help to explain the extraordinary numbers of people with comorbid psychiatric diagnoses (Ross 2000). This common thread of life story is one of the overarching themes of this book – and provides a useful way to maintain focus on the whole.

There are some transdiagnostic approaches that originate in a social science, not biological, understanding of the whole. This includes the Power Threat Meaning (PTM) Framework of The British Psychological Society to address emotional distress using pattern recognition (Johnstone et al. 2018). Post-positivist priorities are also embedded in the salutogenic Sense of Coherence framework that highly values meaningfulness, manageability and comprehensibility and has been taken up by public health systems and primary care clinicians in some parts of the world (Bergh et al. 2006, Nilsson et al. 2003).

Table 3.2 Examples of Transdiagnostic Phenomena

Rumination, Brooding, Negative Thinking	(McEvoy et al. 2013, McLaughlin and Nolen-Hoeksema 2011, Ehring and Watkins 2008)
Perfectionism	(Egan, Wade, and Shafran 2011)
Deficits in Emotion Regulation[2]	(Sloan et al. 2017)
Attentional Control	(Hsu et al. 2015)
Psychological Inflexibility	(Levin et al. 2014)
Heightened Physiological Arousal; Anxiety Sensitivity; Interoceptive Exposure	(Boswell, Farchione, et al. 2013)
Maladaptive Coping Strategies (avoidance, checking, overpreparing); Experiential Avoidance	(Hayes et al. 2004)
Emotional Context Insensitivity	(Coifman and Bonanno 2010)
Suppression	(Magee, Harden, and Teachman 2012)
Compulsivity	(Godier and Park 2014)
Learned Helplessness	(Hiroto and Seligman 1975)
Threat to a Personal Goal	(Linton 2013)
Safety Behaviours	(Nolen-Hoeksema and Watkins 2011)
Intolerance of Uncertainty	(Boswell, Thompson-Hollands, et al. 2013, McEvoy and Erceg-Hurn 2016)
Failure to Regulate	(Linton 2013)

Some thinkers are also considering transdiagnostic processes that impact 'psychobiological factors' (Conway et al. 2018, Egan, Wade, and Shafran 2011, McLaughlin and Nolen-Hoeksema 2011, Kring and Sloan 2009). These also include sleep disturbance (Harvey 2011), dysregulated stress response (Aldi and Pak 2019), neural network abnormalities and neural inflammation (McGorry et al. 2018), and heart rate variability as a biomarker of self-regulation (Beauchaine and Thayer 2015). Those who study the links between emotion and chronic pain name a number of transdiagnostic processes conceptualised as 'failure to regulate'. They see the role of negative emotion and pain as facilitating adaptation to restore homeostasis. They also note the survival importance of context-appropriate responses that are 'in tune' with their environment (Linton 2013).

Each of these approaches to psychological wellbeing is an important step forward – offering an alternative to the current fragmenting approaches to mental health. They add ways to conceptualise Humpty's experience, yet they are not enough to help the practitioner to conceptualise the whole person.

Coherent approaches to the whole matter

Disciplines that are anchored in artificial divisions of the person are still valued more than approaches to seeing the whole. If the many research and practitioner traditions that contribute to understanding the whole person do not learn new ways of conceptualising the whole person, knowledge will continue to be siloed (stored away) in fragments. Useful islands of knowledge culture will not be shared. In the metaphor of the Indonesian islands, beauty and wisdom from islands that are not included or allowed to speak will be left out – this will impoverish the whole. It is also unscientific to claim to offer something comprehensive without considering the whole.

Humpty is a whole that interacts with his world. Science – defined by Ian McGilchrist as 'neither more nor less than patient detailed attention to the world' (McGilchrist 2019, 5) – allows us to observe and interact with that whole. This definition of science does not privilege some forms of knowledge over others. This kind of science notices when something is missing or when we have, as one stakeholder said, 'misnamed' (mhc) something. The pattern watchers – clinicians, patients and researchers – are all observing and learning from, with, or in Humpty. This skill of observing the whole requires a willingness to transcend knowledge and expertise boundaries and to attend to Humpty's context, his relationships, meaning and inner world.

It is difficult for Humpty and those who care for him to maintain an awareness of the whole person. Humpty himself has to integrate different types of knowledge – what transdisciplinary researchers call 'internal perceptions and external information' (McGregor 2018, 192). As discussed in Chapter Two, these perceptions and information require different approaches to understanding. How are these very different forms of knowledge and experience brought together? How do we pay attention to both objective and subjective information in decision-making? What framework should be used to determine what an adequate breadth or scope is? How do we choose a lens that is sufficiently inclusive and considered widely adequate? These questions have deep importance in any consideration of whole person care.

As stated at the outset, this book is written by a generalist who aligns with theoretical and pragmatic transdisciplinary philosophy and practice (Lynch et al. 2020). Transdisciplinary philosophy, with its origins in quantum physics (seeing both the particle and the wave) and hermeneutic phenomenology (seeing the whole and the part) alongside generalism (seeing the complex and the linear), offers wisdom to the practitioner seeking to understand the whole. Complexity science, phenomenology and narrative medicine, as well as clinical pragmatism and critical realism, all also offer some philosophical basis for this work.

The proposed way forward to whole person care will therefore be unashamedly (and unavoidably) generalist and transdisciplinary (Lynch et al. 2020). These philosophical approaches, as outlined in Chapter One, highly value whole person care, relational processes of 'collaborative deliberation' (Elwyn et al. 2014) oriented towards healing, provisional attitudes to knowledge that use integrative wisdom and shared language. They offer a coherent basis for choosing a trade language that helps the islands of knowledge culture to offer a unified approach to Humpty, in his native tongue.

Notes

1 Scientism is "the view that the characteristic inductive methods of the natural sciences are the only source of genuine factual knowledge and, in particular, that they alone can yield true knowledge about man and society" (Bullock and Stallybrass 1999, 775); it is "obsessed with the power and robustness of the natural sciences but ... neglect[s] the suffering human subject and the social context of illness" (Brendel 2007, 312).
2 Emotion regulation: "the set of automatic and controlled processes involved in the initiation, maintenance, and modification of occurrence, intensity, and duration of feeling states" (Webb et al. 2012, 144).

References

Abdi, Reza, and Razieh Pak. 2019. 'The mediating role of emotion dysregulation as a transdiagnostic factor in the relationship between pathological personality dimensions and emotional disorders symptoms severity.' *Personality and Individual Differences* 142: 282–287.

Ajjawi, Rola, and Joy Higgs. 2007. 'Using hermeneutic phenomenology to investigate how experienced practitioners learn to communicate clinical reasoning.' *The Qualitative Report* 12 (4):612–638.

Anandarajah, Gowri. 2008. 'The 3 H and BMSEST models for spirituality in multicultural whole-person medicine.' *The Annals of Family Medicine* 6 (5):448–458.

Anda, R., V. Felitti, J. Bremner, J. Walker, Ch Whitfield, B. Perry, Sh Dube, and W. Giles. 2006. 'The enduring effects of abuse and related adverse experiences in childhood.' *European Archives of Psychiatry and Clinical Neuroscience* 256 (3):174–186. doi:10.1007/s00406-005-0624-4.

Antonovsky, Aaron. 1987. *Unraveling the mystery of health: How people manage stress and stay well.* San Francisco: Jossey-Bass.

Archer, Margaret, Roy Bhaskar, Andrew Collier, Tony Lawson, and Alan Norrie. 2013. *Critical realism: Essential readings.* London: Routledge.

Augsburg, Tanya. 2014. 'Becoming transdisciplinary: The emergence of the transdisciplinary individual.' *World Futures* 70 (3–4):233–247.

Barnacle, Robyn, ed. 2001. *Phenomenology.* Edited by John Bowden, *Qualitative research methods series.* Melbourne: RMIT University Press.

Baxi, U. 2000. 'Transdisciplinarity and transformative praxis.' In *Transdisciplinarity: Recreating integrated knowledge*, edited by M. Somerville, and D. Rapport, 77–85. Oxford: EOLSS.

Beauchaine, Theodore P., and Julian F. Thayer. 2015. 'Heart rate variability as a transdiagnostic biomarker of psychopathology.' *International Journal of Psychophysiology* 98 (2):338–350.

Bergh, Håkan, Amir Baigi, Bengt Fridlund, and Bertil Marklund. 2006. 'Life events, social support and sense of coherence among frequent attenders in primary health care.' *Public Health* 120 (3):229–236.

Bernstein, Jay Hillel. 2015. 'Transdisciplinarity: A review of its origins, development, and current issues.' *Journal of Research Practice* 11 (1):20.

Blundo, Robert. 2001. 'Learning strengths-based practice: Challenging our personal and professional frames.' *Families in Society: The Journal of Contemporary Social Services* 82 (3):296–304.

Boswell, James F., Todd J. Farchione, Shannon Sauer-Zavala, Heather W. Murray, Meghan R. Fortune, and David H. Barlow. 2013. 'Anxiety sensitivity and interoceptive exposure: A transdiagnostic construct and change strategy.' *Behavior Therapy* 44 (3):417–431.

Boswell, James F., Johanna Thompson-Hollands, Todd J. Farchione, and David H. Barlow. 2013. 'Intolerance of uncertainty: A common factor in the treatment of emotional disorders.' *Journal of Clinical Psychology* 69 (6):630–645.

Bowlby, John. 1977. 'The making and breaking of affectional bonds. I. Aetiology and psychopathology in the light of attachment theory. An expanded version of the Fiftieth Maudsley Lecture, delivered before the Royal College of Psychiatrists, 19 November 1976.' *The British Journal of Psychiatry* 130 (3):201–210.

Brendel, David H. 2007. 'Beyond Engel: Clinical pragmatism as the foundation of psychiatric practice.' *Philosophy, Psychiatry, & Psychology* 14 (4):311–313.

Browne, Annette J., Colleen M. Varcoe, Sabrina T. Wong, Victoria L. Smye, Josée Lavoie, Doreen Littlejohn, David Tu, Olive Godwin, Murry Krause, and Koushambhi B. Khan. 2012. 'Closing the health equity gap: Evidence-based strategies for primary health care organizations.' *International Journal for Equity in Health* 11 (1):1–15.

Buckholtz, Joshua W., and Andreas Meyer-Lindenberg. 2012. 'Psychopathology and the human connectome: Toward a transdiagnostic model of risk for mental illness.' *Neuron* 74 (6):990–1004.

Bullock, Alan, and Oliver Stallybrass. 1999. *The new Fontana dictionary of modern thought.* London: HarperCollins Publishers Limited.

Butler, Emily A., and Ashley K. Randall. 2013. 'Emotional coregulation in close relationships.' *Emotion Review* 5 (2):202–210.

Casey, P., C. Dowrick, and G. Wilkinson. 2001. 'Adjustment disorders fault line in the psychiatric glossary.' *The British Journal of Psychiatry* 179 (6):479–481.

Cassidy, Jude, and Phillip R. Shaver. 1999. *Handbook of attachment: Theory, research, and clinical applications.* New York: The Guildford Press.

Charon, Rita. 2006. *Narrative medicine: Honoring the stories of illness.* Oxford: Oxford University Press.

Christie, Michael. 2006. 'Transdisciplinary research and aboriginal knowledge.' *The Australian Journal of Indigenous Education* 35:78–89. https://doi.org/10.1017/S13260 11100004191.

Coifman, Karin G., and George A. Bonanno. 2010. 'When distress does not become depression: Emotion context sensitivity and adjustment to bereavement.' *Journal of Abnormal Psychology* 119 (3):479–490.

Conway, Christopher C., Elizabeth B. Raposa, Constance Hammen, and Patricia A. Brennan. 2018. 'Transdiagnostic pathways from early social stress to psychopathology: A 20-year prospective study.' *Journal of Child Psychology and Psychiatry* 59 (8):855–862.

Cosco, Theodore D., Kenneth Howse, and Carol Brayne. 2017. 'Healthy ageing, resilience and wellbeing.' *Epidemiology and Psychiatric Sciences* 26 (6):579–583.

Courtois, C., and J. Ford. 2014. *Into the Whirlwind: Clinical and scientific innovations in the treatment of complex Trauma.* Melbourne.

Cuthbert, Bruce N., and Thomas R. Insel. 2013. Toward the future of psychiatric diagnosis: The seven pillars of RDoC. *BMC Medicine* 11 (126). Accessed 15/10/16. https://doi.org /10.1186/1741-7015-11-126.

Dewar, Belinda, and Mike Nolan. 2013. 'Caring about caring: Developing a model to implement compassionate relationship centred care in an older people care setting.' *International Journal of Nursing Studies* 50 (9):1247–1258.

Donner-Banzhoff, Norbert. 2018. 'Solving the diagnostic challenge: A patient-centered approach.' *The Annals of Family Medicine* 16 (4):353–358.

Dowrick, Christopher. 2009. 'When diagnosis fails: A commentary on McPherson & Armstrong.' *Social Science & Medicine* 69 (8):1144–1146.

Dowrick, Christopher, Carl May, Michael Richardson, and Peter Bundred. 1996. 'The biopsychosocial model of general practice: Rhetoric or reality?' *British Journal of General Practice* 46:105–107.

Egan, Sarah J., Tracey D. Wade, and Roz Shafran. 2011. 'Perfectionism as a transdiagnostic process: A clinical review.' *Clinical Psychology Review* 31 (2):203–212.

Ehring, Thomas, and Edward R. Watkins. 2008. 'Repetitive negative thinking as a transdiagnostic process.' *International Journal of Cognitive Therapy* 1 (3):192–205.

Elwyn, G., A. Lloyd, C. May, T. van der Weijden, A. Stiggelbout, A. Edwards, D.L.T. Frosch, T. Rapley, T. Barr Walsh, S.W. Grande, V. Montori, and R. Epstein. 2014. 'Collaborative deliberation: A model for patient care.' *Patient Education and Counselling* 97 (2):158–164. https://doi.org/10.1016/j.pec.2014.07.027.

Engel, G.L. 1977. 'The need for a new medical model: A challenge for biomedicine.' *Science* 196 (4286):129–136.

Enns, Carolyn Zerbe, Jean Campbell, Christine A. Courtois, Michael C. Gottlieb, Karen P. Lese, Mary S. Gilbert, and Linda Forrest. 1998. 'Working with adult clients who may have experienced childhood abuse: Recommendations for assessment and practice.' *Professional Psychology: Research and Practice* 29 (3):245–256.

Felitti, V.J., R.F. Anda, D. Nordenberg, D.F. Williamson, A.M. Spitz, V. Edwards, M.P. Koss, and J.S. Marks. 1998. 'Relationship of childhood abuse and household dysfunction to many of the leading causes of death in adults: The Adverse Childhood Experiences (ACE) study.' *American Journal of Preventive Medicine* 14 (4):245–258.

Fisher, Janina. 2011. 'Sensorimotor approaches to trauma treatment.' *Advances in Psychiatric Treatment* 17 (3):171–177.

Forgeard, Marie J.C., Emily A.P. Haigh, Aaron T. Beck, Richard J. Davidson, Fritz A. Henn, Steven F. Maier, Helen S. Mayberg, and Martin E.P. Seligman. 2011. 'Beyond depression: Toward a process-based approach to research, diagnosis, and treatment.' *Clinical Psychology: Science and Practice* 18 (4):275–299.

Gee, G., P. Dudgeon, C. Schultz, A. Hart, and K. Kelly. 2014. 'Aboriginal and Torres Strait Islander social and emotional wellbeing.' In *Working together: Aboriginal and Torres Strait Islander mental health and wellbeing principles and practice*, edited by P. Dudgeon, H. Milroy, and R. Walker, 55–68. Canberra: Commonwealth of Australia. https://www.telethonkids.org.au/globalassets/media/documents/aboriginal-health/working-together-second-edition/working-together-aboriginal-and-wellbeing-2014.pdf

Ghaemi, S. Nassir. 2007. 'Existence and pluralism: The rediscovery of Karl Jaspers.' *Psychopathology* 40:75–82.

Ghaemi, S. Nassir 2009. 'The rise and fall of the biopsychosocial model.' *The British Journal of Psychiatry* 195 (1):3–4.

Gibbs, Paul. 2015. 'Transdisciplinarity as epistemology, ontology or principles of practical judgement.' In *Transdisciplinary professional learning and practice*, edited by P. Gibbs, 151–164. Cham: Springer.

Godier, Lauren R., and Rebecca J. Park. 2014. 'Compulsivity in anorexia nervosa: A transdiagnostic concept.' *Frontiers in Psychology* 5:778. https://doi.org/10.3389/fpsyg.2014.00778.

Goldberg, David. 1992. 'A classification of psychological distress for use in primary care settings.' *Social Science & Medicine* 35 (2):189–193.

Gray, Barbara. 2008. 'Enhancing transdisciplinary research through collaborative leadership.' *American Journal of Preventive Medicine* 35 (2):S124–S132.

Hagedorn, Rosemary. 1992. *Occupational therapy: Foundations for practice: Models, frames of reference and core skills.* Edinburgh: Churchill Livingstone.

Haggerty, G., M.J. Hilsenroth, and R. Vala-Stewart. 2009. 'Attachment and interpersonal distress: Examining the relationship between attachment styles and interpersonal problems in a clinical population.' *Clinical Psychology & Psychotherapy* 16:1–9. doi: 10.1002/cpp.

Hamberger, E. 2004. 'Transdisciplinarity: A scientific essential.' *Annals of the New York Academy of Sciences* 1028:487–496. doi:10.1196/annals.1322.039.

Harris, Mark, Sarah Dennis, and Megan Pillay. 2013. 'Multimorbidity: Negotiating priorities and making progress.' *Australian Family Physician* 42 (12):850–854.

Harvey, Allison G., Greg Murray, Rebecca A. Chandler, and Adriane Soehner. 2011. 'Sleep disturbance as transdiagnostic: consideration of neurobiological mechanisms.' *Clinical Psychology Review* 31(2): 225–235.

Hayes, Steven C., Kirk Strosahl, Kelly G. Wilson, Richard T. Bissett, Jacqueline Pistorello, Dosheen Toarmino, Melissa A. Polusny, Thane A. Dykstra, Sonja V. Batten, and John Bergan. 2004. 'Measuring experiential avoidance: A preliminary test of a working model.' *The Psychological Record* 54 (4):553–578.

Healy, Karen. 2014. *Social work theories in context: Creating frameworks for practice.* 2nd ed. China: Palgrave Macmillan.

Hiroto, Donald S., and Martin E. Seligman. 1975. 'Generality of learned helplessness in man.' *Journal of Personality and Social Psychology* 31 (2):311–327.

Hsu, Kean J., Courtney Beard, Lara Rifkin, Daniel G. Dillon, Diego A. Pizzagalli, and Thröstur Björgvinsson. 2015. 'Transdiagnostic mechanisms in depression and anxiety: The role of rumination and attentional control.' *Journal of Affective Disorders* 188:22–27.

Hutchinson, T.A. 2011. *Whole person care : A new paradigm for the 21st century.* New York: Springer.

Johansen, May-Lill, and Mette Bech Risor. 2017. 'What is the problem with medically unexplained symptoms for GPs? A meta-synthesis of qualitative studies.' *Patient Education and Counseling* 100 (4):647–654.

Johnstone, L., M. Boyle, J. Cromby, J. Dillon, D. Harper, P. Kinderman, E. Longden, D. Pilgrim, and J. Read. 2018. *The power threat meaning framework: Towards the identification of patterns in emotional distress, unusual experiences and troubled or troubling behaviour, as an alternative to functional psychiatric diagnosis.* Leicester British Psychological Society.

Kate, M.-A., and M. Dorahy. 2019. 'Complex trauma disorders.' In *Humanising mental health in Australia: A guide to Trauma- informed approaches,* edited by R. Benjamin, J. Haliburn, and S. King, 84–97. London: Routledge Taylor and Francis Group.

Kirkengen, Anna Luise. 2010. *The lived experience of violation: How abused children become unhealthy adults.* Vol. 1. Bucharest: Zeta Books.

Kirkengen, Anna Luise, Tor-Johan Ekeland, Linn Getz, Irene Hetlevik, Edvin Schei, Elling Ulvestad and Arne Johan Vetlesen. 2016. 'Medicine's perception of reality–a split picture: Critical reflections on apparent anomalies within the biomedical theory of science.' *Journal of Evaluation in Clinical Practice* 22 (4):496–501.

Kirkengen, Anna Luise, Bente Prytz Mjolstad, Linn Getz, Elling Ulvestad, and Irene Hetlevik. 2014. 'Can person-free medical knowledge inform person-centered medical practice.' *European Journal for Person Centered Healthcare* 2:32–36.

Kirkengen, Anna Luise, and Eline Thornquist. 2012. 'The lived body as a medical topic: An argument for an ethically informed epistemology.' *Journal of Evaluation in Clinical Practice* 18 (5):1095–1101.

Klein, Julie Thompson. 2015. 'Reprint of "Discourses of transdisciplinarity: Looking back to the future".' *Futures* 65:10–16.

Kotov, Roman, Robert F. Krueger, David Watson, Thomas M. Achenbach, Robert R. Althoff, R. Michael Bagby, Timothy A. Brown, William T. Carpenter, Avshalom Caspi, and Lee Anna Clark. 2017. 'The hierarchical taxonomy of psychopathology (HiTOP): A dimensional alternative to traditional nosologies.' *Journal of Abnormal Psychology* 126 (4):454–477.

Kring, Ann M., and Denise M. Sloan. 2009. *Emotion regulation and psychopathology: A transdiagnostic approach to etiology and treatment.* New York, NY: Guilford Press.

Krueger, Robert F., and Nicholas R. Eaton. 2015. 'Transdiagnostic factors of mental disorders.' *World Psychiatry* 14 (1):27–29.

Levin, Michael E., Chelsea MacLane, Susan Daflos, John R. Seeley, Steven C. Hayes, Anthony Biglan, and Jacqueline Pistorello. 2014. 'Examining psychological inflexibility as a transdiagnostic process across psychological disorders.' *Journal of Contextual Behavioral Science* 3 (3):155–163.

Lewis, Bradley. 2006. *Moving beyond Prozac, DSM, and the new psychiatry: The birth of postpsychiatry.* Ann Arbour: University of Michigan Press.

Lewis, Bradley. 2014. 'The four Ps, narrative psychiatry, and the story of George Engel.' *Philosophy, Psychiatry, & Psychology* 21 (3):195–197.

Linton, Steven J. 2013. 'A transdiagnostic approach to pain and emotion.' *Journal of Applied Biobehavioral Research* 18 (2):82–103.

Low, Douglas. 2010. 'Merleau-Ponty and a reconsideration of alienation.' *Philosophy Today* 54 (2):199–211.

Lynch, J.M. 2019. *Sense of safety: A whole person approach to distress.* PhD, Primary Care Clinical Unit, University of Queensland.

Lynch, J.M., D.A. Askew, G.K. Mitchell, and K.L. Hegarty. 2012. 'Beyond symptoms: Defining primary care mental health clinical assessment priorities, content and process.' *Social Science & Medicine* 74 (2):143–9. doi:10.1016/j.socscimed.2011.08.043.

Lynch, J.M., C.F. Dowrick, Pamela Meredith, S.L.T. McGregor, and Mieke Van Driel. 2020. 'Transdisciplinary generalism: Naming the epistemology and philosophy of the generalist.' *Journal of Evaluation in Clinical Practice*, 1–10.

Lyotard, Jean-François. 1984. *The postmodern condition: A report on knowledge.* Vol. 10. Minneapolis: University of Minnesota Press.

Maercker, Andreas, Chris R. Brewin, Richard A. Bryant, Marylene Cloitre, Geoffrey M. Reed, Mark van Ommeren, Asma Humayun, Lynne M. Jones, Ashraf Kagee, and Augusto E. Llosa. 2013. 'Proposals for mental disorders specifically associated with stress in the International Classification of Diseases-11.' *The Lancet* 381 (9878):1683–1685.

Magee, Joshua C., K. Paige Harden, and Bethany A. Teachman. 2012. 'Psychopathology and thought suppression: A quantitative review.' *Clinical Psychology Review* 32 (3):189–201.

Martin, C.M. 2003. 'Making a case for transdisciplinarity.' *Canadian Family Physician* 49 (7):905–906.

Maxwell, J.A. 2002. 'Understanding and validity in qualitative research.' In *The qualitative researcher's companion*, edited by A.M. Huberman, and M.B. Miles, 37–64. California: Sage Publications.

McEvoy, Peter M., and David M. Erceg-Hurn. 2016. 'The search for universal transdiagnostic and trans-therapy change processes: Evidence for intolerance of uncertainty.' *Journal of Anxiety Disorders* 41:96–107.

McEvoy, Peter M., Hunna Watson, Edward R. Watkins, and Paula Nathan. 2013. 'The relationship between worry, rumination, and comorbidity: Evidence for repetitive negative thinking as a transdiagnostic construct.' *Journal of Affective Disorders* 151 (1):313–320.

McEwen, Bruce S. 2007. 'Physiology and neurobiology of stress and adaptation: Central role of the brain.' *Physiological Reviews* 87 (3):873–904.

McGilchrist, Iain. 2019. *The master and his emissary: The divided brain and the making of the Western world*. London: Yale University Press.

McGorry, Patrick D., Jessica A. Hartmann, Rachael Spooner, and Barnaby Nelson. 2018. 'Beyond the "at risk mental state" concept: Transitioning to transdiagnostic psychiatry.' *World Psychiatry* 17 (2):133–142.

McGregor, S.L. 2004. The nature of transdisciplinary research and practice. Kappa Omicron Nu human sciences working paper series.

McGregor, S.L.T. 2011. 'Transdisciplinary axiology: To be or not to be.' *Integral Leadership Review* 11 (3). http://integralleadershipreview.com/2011/08/transdisciplinary-axiology-to-be-or-not-to-be

McGregor, S.L.T. 2015. 'Transdisciplinary knowledge creation.' In *Transdisciplinary professional learning and practice*, edited by P. Gibbs, 9–24. New York: Springer.

McGregor, S.L.T. 2017. *Understanding and evaluating research: A critical guide*. Online: SAGE Publications.

McGregor, S.L.T. 2018. 'Philosophical underpinnings of the transdisciplinary research methodology.' *Transdisciplinary Journal of Engineering and Science* 9:182–198.

McLaughlin, Katie A., and Susan Nolen-Hoeksema. 2011. 'Rumination as a transdiagnostic factor in depression and anxiety.' *Behaviour Research and Therapy* 49 (3):186–193.

McWhinney, Ian R. 1964. *The early signs of illness: Observations in general practice*. London: Pitman Thomas Nelson.

Mezzich, Juan E., Ihsan M. Salloum, C. Robert Cloninger, Luis Salvador-Carulla, Laurence J. Kirmayer, Claudio E.M. Banzato, Jan Wallcraft, and Michel Botbol. 2010. 'Person-centred integrative diagnosis: Conceptual bases and structural model.' *The Canadian Journal of Psychiatry* 55 (11):701–708.

Mezzich, Juan E., Jon Snaedal, Chris Van Weel, and Iona Heath. 2010. 'Toward person-centered medicine: From disease to patient to person.' *Mount Sinai Journal of Medicine: A Journal of Translational and Personalized Medicine: A Journal of Translational and Personalized Medicine* 77 (3):304–306.

Moos, Rudolf H. 1984. 'Context and coping: Toward a unifying conceptual framework.' *American Journal of Community Psychology* 12 (1):5–36.

Moser, Susanne, Sara Meerow, James Arnott, and Emily Jack-Scott. 2019. 'The turbulent world of resilience: Interpretations and themes for transdisciplinary dialogue.' *Climatic Change* 153 (1–2):21–40.

Neimeyer, Robert A. 2001. *Meaning reconstruction & the experience of loss*. Washington, DC: American Psychological Association.

Nicolescu, Basarab, and Atila Ertas. 2013. *Transdisciplinary theory and practice*. Texas: The ATLAS Publishing.

Nicolescu, Basarab, E. Morin, and L. de Freitas. 1994. *The charter of transdisciplinarity*. First World Congress on transdisciplinarity, Convento de Arrabida, Portugal.

Nilsson, Berit, Lars Holmgren, Birgitta Stegmayr, and Göran Westman. 2003. 'Sense of coherence-stability over time and relation to health, disease, and psychosocial changes in a general population: A longitudinal study.' *Scandinavian Journal of Public Health* 31 (4):297–304.

NIMH. 2020. 'RDoC constructs.' *NIMH.* Accessed 15/2/20. https://www.nimh.nih.gov/research/research-funded-by-nimh/rdoc/constructs/rdoc-matrix.shtml.

Nolen-Hoeksema, Susan, and Edward R. Watkins. 2011. 'A heuristic for developing transdiagnostic models of psychopathology: Explaining multifinality and divergent trajectories.' *Perspectives on Psychological Science* 6 (6):589–609.

Ogden, P., K. Minton, and C. Pain, eds. 2006. *Trauma and the body. A sensorimotor approach to psychotherapy.* New York: W.W. Norton and Company Inc.

Park, Crystal L. 2010. 'Making sense of the meaning literature: An integrative review of meaning making and its effects on adjustment to stressful life events.' *Psychological Bulletin* 136 (2):257–301.

Polk, Merritt. 2014. 'Achieving the promise of transdisciplinarity: A critical exploration of the relationship between transdisciplinary research and societal problem solving.' *Sustainability Science* 9 (4):439–451.

Porges, S.W. 2011. *The polyvagal theory: Neurophysiological foundations of emotions, attachment, communication, and self-regulation.* New York: WW Norton & Company.

Reeve, Joanne 2010. 'Interpretive medicine: Supporting generalism in a changing primary care world.' *Occasional Paper Royal College of General Practitioners* 88:1–20.

Reeve, Joanne. 2018. 'Primary care redesign for person-centred care: Delivering an international generalist revolution.' *Australian Journal of Primary Health* 24 (4):330–336.

Reeve, Joanne, C Dowrick, F.G.K. Freeman, J. Gunn, F. Mair, C. May, S. Mercer, V. Palmer, A. Howe, and G. Irving. 2013. 'Examining the practice of generalist expertise: A qualitative study identifying constraints and solutions.' *JRSM Short Reports* 4 (12):1–9.

Reuben, David B., and Mary E. Tinetti. 2012. 'Goal-oriented patient care – an alternative health outcomes paradigm.' *New England Journal of Medicine* 366 (9):777–779.

Ross, Colin A. 2000. *The trauma model: A solution to the problem of comorbidity in psychiatry.* Richardson, TX: Manitou Communications.

Sadler, J.Z., and Y.F. Hulgus. 1992. 'Clinical problem solving and the biopsychosocial model.' *The American Journal of Psychiatry* 149 (10):1315–1323.

Sauer-Zavala, Shannon, Cassidy A. Gutner, Todd J. Farchione, Hannah T. Boettcher, Jacqueline R. Bullis, and David H. Barlow. 2017. 'Current definitions of "transdiagnostic" in treatment development: A search for consensus.' *Behavior Therapy* 48 (1):128–138.

Schiøtz, M.L., et al. 2017. 'Social disparities in the prevalence of multimorbidity–a register-based population study.' *BMC Public Health* 17 (1):422.

Schore, A.N. 1996. 'The experience-dependent maturation of a regulatory system in the orbital prefrontal cortex and the origin of developmental psychopathology.' *Development and Psychopathology* 8:59–88.

Skinner, Ellen A., and Melanie J. Zimmer-Gembeck. 2007. 'The development of coping.' *Annual Review of Psychology* 58:119–144.

Sloan, Elise, Kate Hall, Richard Moulding, Shayden Bryce, Helen Mildred and Petra K. Staiger. 2017. 'Emotion regulation as a transdiagnostic treatment construct across anxiety, depression, substance, eating and borderline personality disorders: A systematic review.' *Clinical Psychology Review* 57:141–163.

Stange, Kurt C., William L. Miller, and I. McWhinney. 2001. 'Developing the knowledge base of family practice.' *Family Medicine* 33 (4):286–297.

Sturmberg, Joachim P., Jeanette M. Bennett, Carmel M. Martin, and Martin Picard. 2017. '"Multimorbidity" as the manifestation of network disturbances.' *Journal of Evaluation in Clinical Practice* 23 (1):199–208.

Thomas, Hayley, Megan Best, and Geoffrey Mitchell. 2020. 'Whole-person care in general practice: "The nature of whole-person care".' *Australian Journal of General Practice* 49 (1/2):54–60. doi: 10.31128/AJGP-05-19-49501.

Waterman, G Scott. 2014. 'Formulation as diagnosis: Toward a post-DSM, post-biopsychosocial world.' *Philosophy, Psychiatry, & Psychology* 21 (3):211–213.

Webb, Thomas L., Eleanor Miles, and Paschal Sheeran. 2012. 'Dealing with feeling: a meta-analysis of the effectiveness of strategies derived from the process model of emotion regulation.' *Psychological Bulletin* 138 (4): 775.

Windle, Gill, and Robert T. Woods. 2004. 'Variations in subjective wellbeing: The mediating role of a psychological resource.' *Ageing & Society* 24 (4):583–602.

Wing, J.K., A.S. Beevor, R.H. Curtis, S.G.B. Park, J. Hadden, and A. Burns. 1998. 'Health of the nation outcome scales (HoNOS): Research and development.' *The British Journal of Psychiatry* 172 (1):11–18.

4   Why *sense of safety*? A strengths-based approach to the whole

- *Sense of safety* gives comfort and courage
- *Sense of safety* is trauma informed and strengths based
- *Sense of safety* is built within relationships
- *Sense of safety* is a physiological reality
- *Sense of safety* is a *gestalt* whole person experience

One day I asked a severe childhood trauma and neglect survivor I had cared for over years if there was anywhere in her childhood she felt safe. She has kindly shared her answer: 'On the school bus'.

Neither home nor school felt safe. As a child, she only felt safe for the few minutes she was on the school bus, weekdays and school days. In the rest of her life she was trapped in vigilance, terror, confusion, loneliness or pain. We know that this kind of chronic threat is not uncommon in our communities, and it impacts lifelong wellbeing, including physiological health (Felitti et al. 1998). When I asked her what it felt like to be on the bus, she said: 'It was like a deep breath'.

The physicality of her answer struck me as did her vivid memory of that safety years later. As a biomedically trained doctor, I imagined her on that bus having a few moments of reprieve. I imagined her breathing and heart rate slowing and her muscles relaxing for a few moments. I wondered how her endocrine and immune systems responded to this reprieve. With her, years later, those moments to take her breath were a resource, a memory of something good in her life, a tiny window into a world of what is possible away from deprivation and abuse.

I looked through that window too. My clinical work with adult survivors of childhood trauma and neglect showed me the many and varied ways that safety can be threatened – from crowded living arrangements to inner despair, from invasion to disconnection. They showed me how much *sense of safety* changed capacity to think straight, to trust others and to feel calm. I became a Bowerbird searching for research evidence about safety. I found evidence in the literature on trauma and attachment, psychophysiology, developmental paediatrics, couple therapy, attention, immunology, endocrinology, emotion and interpersonal neurobiology. I also found evidence in the social deprivation, built environment and food and water security literature. *Sense of safety* is important in many parts of the whole.

So, I became a clinician searching for safety in my patients' lives. I changed my assessment priorities. I paid more attention to body movement, tone of voice and silences. I learned how to facilitate emotion regulation during story telling in my consultation room and how to be careful using words that may trigger flashbacks in the other person. I attended to people, places, hobbies, spirituality, favourite recipes, tastes and smells, memories, music, books or pets in each person's life story that might be a window out of a survival mode and into a *sense of safety*. Sensing you are safe – for a moment – for a window of your day – makes healing and restoration possible. Sensing you are safe is a fundamental element of wellbeing of the whole person.

Those who have been the most traumatised, those who care for them clinically and those who research trauma have clearly shown the importance of safety to normal development, relationships and physiology. They have also revealed the growth that can happen when you feel safe. This is the clinical and research background to the idea of using the ordinary English phrase 'sense of safety' to assess distress and build wellbeing. As one stakeholder said: 'Safety: this is it, this is the treatment, this is your job, it's not just a complication' (mhc).

Sense of safety: A whole person approach

Psychophysiologist Stephen Porges asserts: 'the goal of civilisation is to be safe in someone else's arms' (Porges 2014, audio). He names our mammalian need for one another in order to have moments when we are immobile and yet not on guard, allowing restorative rest, reproduction and lactation. Decades earlier, Maslow called the human organism 'safety-seeking' (Maslow 1954, 1818) and named safety as a human meta-need (Maslow 1954, 8) of the 'integrated organised whole' (Maslow 1954, 3). Attachment, trauma and stress research have confirmed the impact of relational, psychological and physical stressors across the lifespan on neurology, metabolism, immunity, inner experience and sense of self (Lynch and Kirkengen 2019, Slavich et al. 2010, Schore 2001). At a physiological level and a relational level, we need safety for health.

There are other words that imply a *sense of safety* as a physiological whole person experience, such as calm, rest, relaxed, at ease and 'home-like being in the world' (Svenaeus 2001, 193). The related terms 'felt security' (Maunder and Hunter 2001) and 'sense of security' (Milberg et al. 2014) are already used in medical settings. The term 'psychological safety' is used in workplace team functioning and learning (Carmeli, Brueller, and Dutton 2009) to describe 'a climate in which people are comfortable being (and expressing) themselves' (Edmondson 2004, 240). The actual words 'sense of safety' are already used in the built environment literature – signifying a home with a sense of solidarity with neighbours and green spaces around it (Kuo, Bacaicoa, and Sullivan 1998). Coming from a Danish word meaning 'to give courage, comfort, joy' (2019), the now international word *hygge* includes experiences of contentment, cosiness, wellness and comfortable connection. As we will discover in later chapters, *sense of safety* includes these relational and physical experiences that give both comfort and courage.

The concept of *sense of safety* as a clinical theme or pattern to recognise in the whole person will be examined throughout this book. A key support for this assertion that *sense of safety* is wholeness is the Latin root of the word safe – linked to the word *salvus*, which is related to the concepts of *salus* ('good health'), *saluber* ('healthful') and *solidus* ('solid'). All of these words are derived from the Proto-Indo-European base word *solwos*, meaning 'whole'. This is the central tenet of this book – that *sense of safety* is central to wellbeing, can help us to see the whole person and help them become well – to become whole.

Sense of safety: **Trauma-informed and strengths-based**

Thankfully, the words 'trauma-informed' and 'trauma-specific' care have become more well known in the community. Those who have a lived experience of trauma and the practitioners who care for them have finally had their voices heard: life story, meaning, relationships and experiences of threat impact wellbeing. I therefore see that the term 'trauma-informed' is a gift to those who have sought to bring awareness to the complexity of lived experience and distress – it is a shorthand that brings attention to more than biological or psychiatric ways of framing distress. When I teach generalists, I say that trauma-informed care is in effect a code for another way of seeing the world – one where relationships, sense of self, meaning and life story (not just bodily experiences) are part of understanding health and caring for the whole.

The trauma literature also has an explicit goal of safety. Writers speak of the importance of establishing a 'sense of safety and stability' (Enns et al. 1998, 248) in trauma-informed therapy that includes capacity for affect regulation, a sense of mastery, capacity to cope and strengthened social relationships. Key trauma-informed clinicians speak of the therapeutic goals of restoration of a 'visceral sense of control and safety' (Van Der Kolk 2014b, 31). They assert that people present for help because they have lost the capacity to 'feel safe with other human beings, or even with themselves' (Frewen et al. 2015, xiv).

Christine Courtois and Julian Ford (2009) note altered perception and trust in relationship to self, others, meaning, consciousness and connection to body as a result of chronic threat. There are also objective signs of *sense of safety* available to practitioners as they notice posture, breathing, prosody, self-acceptance, capacity to express emotion, capacity for insight and reduced defensiveness (Rappoport 1997, 253). Safety is one of the five key principles listed in international guidelines for trauma-informed care. The other principles are choice, collaboration, empowerment and trustworthiness (Kezelman and Stavropoulos 2012), which I would see as part of building *sense of safety*. Geller and Porges (2014, 188) declare that 'client safety … [is] a core prerequisite for effective therapeutic work regardless of the therapeutic approach'. This endorsement of the clinical importance of safety is relevant for any discipline that encounters distressed people – including the primary care setting.

As well as being a gift – raising awareness of the whole person experience – the concept of trauma has some limitations in ways that 'trauma' can be interpreted. It can limit how wide we look (missing neglect or overwhelming adult experiences); it can be viewed as only relevant if there is physical injury or risk of physical injury; it can have connotations of facilitating victimhood or dwelling on dark times in the past.

I once cared for a lady who had terrible flashbacks in her seventies to a time in her primary school years where she played hide and seek in a cupboard and she could not get out (and no one noticed her absence and came looking for her). She feared that she would die in that cupboard. I learned that what is traumatic is a subjective internal experience. Traumatic experiences can be imagined, remembered, relived. They could be about our bodies, or our identities, or our relationships, about existential beliefs, about our homes, keepsakes, livelihoods and even our pets. For example, people can be traumatised by loss of identity as a productive worker (through injury or retirement), or loss of identity as mother (through miscarriage, stillbirth, abortion, death or estrangement of children at any age), or loss of identity as beautiful or strong (through disfigurement, demeaning words, illness or disability) or even loss of identity as child (by being given overwhelming responsibility – as in children who are parentified by an unwell or neglectful parent). They can be traumatised by loss from shattered assumptions (Janoff-Bulman 1985), loss of imagined success or loss of life partner (Christakis and Iwashyna 2003). Fear of the unknown and uncertainty are also significant stressors to human beings (Carleton 2016a, 2016b). Complicated or maladaptive grief is marked by evidence of overwhelm with symptoms of avoidance, intrusive memories and failure to adapt to loss (Horowitz et al. 2003). As Margret Tomasdotttir (2016, 2) notes: 'it is *subjective experience,* not quantifiable events, that become biologically inscribed' (original author's italics) – this is relevant for whole person care. The word 'trauma' unfortunately can mean these less visible causes of distress become disenfranchised.[1] All forms of threat need to be addressed in any generalist framework developed to address distress. A wide view – sensitive to any cause of *loss of sense of safety* might enfranchise all these varied forms of loss.

The physical implications of the word 'trauma' can also be a limitation. In the emergency department, 'trauma' usually means dramatic physical impact or lacerations often involving life-threatening loss of blood that requires surgery or urgent medical care. This kind of trauma requires airlifts to hospital and draws funding for treatment centres and research. Even in the psychiatric use of the word, in the diagnosis of Post Traumatic Stress Disorder emerging from the Vietnam War, its original definition was linked directly to actual physical events – having had (or witnessed) life-threatening events (by which they meant physical body-threatening). This field of research and practice has remained very positivist in its definitions of observable or threatened physical trauma.

Although a misunderstanding of the term, the term 'trauma-informed' can also be constrained by understandings that see it as a way to define a person who has been a victim in their life. It can be seen as a mode of treatment that only focuses on 'unpacking Pandora's box' without skills to treat it, as one GP warily said to me. Clinicians can be wary of learning about people's life stories or screening for trauma if they think it is only looking at the past in a way that might cause harm and distress without any clear idea what to do next. The word trauma can also cause internal distress for those who live in the double bind of attachment to their perpetrator (Ross 2000) and therefore do not want to blame anyone or label any-one as abusive, leaving them with no option but to minimise their need for help. These limitations can prevent appropriate referrals or treatment.

Assessing *sense of safety* is a strength-based approach to any subjective or objec-tive trauma or threat. It offers a clear way forward – a healing goal that can guide assessment, therapeutic process and direction. This can guide content and relational processes of therapy. It can be a shared process of appraisal, aligning practitioners with Humpty's innate priorities and language. It can even guide the moment-by-moment safety during history taking: safety takes precedence over story (Courtois 2004, 416). As a lay term or ordinary phrase, *sense of safety* can also enfranchise ordinary non-professional approaches to healing. It means that Humpty, and all the practitioners that care for him in any field, can offer relational safety and simple human kindnesses that build *sense of safety* (Allen 2013). *Sense of safety* and *loss of sense of safety* (as will be discussed in Chapter Five) are therefore concepts that can integrate the whole person gift of trauma-informed care while mitigating its limitations.

The concept of *sense of safety* integrates the science and therapeutic insights from the trauma-informed community with a strengths-based, goal-oriented approach. The goal is to build *sense of safety* in many aspects of the person's life. The literature on post traumatic growth is a helpful way to understand the purpose of trauma-informed care – seeing your own strengths, who you can trust and how to understand your world (Calhoun and Tedeschi 2006). One of the original writers to identify traumatic experiences in women in their close rela-tionships, Judith Herman, identified three stages of trauma-informed treatment. She named the first stage 'establishment of safety', the second as 'remembrance and mourning' and the third as 'reconnection with ordinary life' (Herman 2015). These form the basis for what is still seen as the gold standard for treatment in the trauma-informed literature. The first phase is now known as 'Stabilisation', the second as 'Processing' and the third as 'Integration' (Kezelman and Stavropoulos 2019, Kezelman and Stavropoulos 2012). Seen through a *sense of safety* lens and aligning with Herman's original descriptions, these tasks are seen less as phases and more as interacting processes requiring *sense of safety* at every stage. These strength-based, trauma-informed *sense of safety goals of care* are named in Figure 4.1 alongside the names for each stage proposed by Hermans (1992) and current trauma-informed guidelines (Stavropolous 2019).

Sense of safety: Built within relationships

The attachment field of literature reveals the importance of caring relationships to signal safety at a neurological level (Eisenberger et al. 2011) and offer expe-riences of 'felt security' (Allen and Manning 2007, 30). This security includes

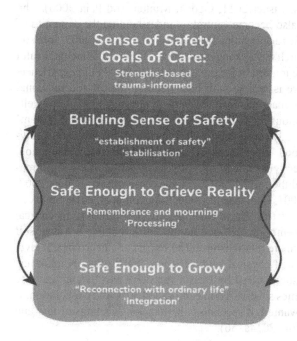

Figure 4.1 Strengths-based trauma-informed *sense of safety goals of care*: integrating concepts.

attuned relational experiences of both 'safe haven' (providing soothing comfort and refuge) and 'secure base' (encouraging capacity to engage with the world and take appropriate risks to step out and explore, learn and grow) (Kerns et al. 2015). This literature is used extensively in therapeutic and parenting training settings as described in the Circle of Security intervention (Powell et al. 2013). This attachment literature has changed my day-to-day clinical work by helping me to see the fears of each person and the relational healing safety that can be a gift of the therapeutic relationship. Loneliness researchers also point to the healing and physical health impacts of connection (Murthy 2020). Attachment research is a key foundation of the concept of *sense of safety*.

Attachment research grew out of the observations of patterns of parent-child interactions that they framed as varying levels of capacity to safely 'attach' or bond (or feel safe) with each other (Bowlby 1979). Bowlby's observations that nurturing and attachment were lifelong and healthy were initially disregarded by the medical establishment (Rutter 1995). His work with Mary Ainsworth, building on Blatz's 'security theory' (Blatz 1973), has transformed approaches to early childhood and parenting. This area of research expanded into the study of neurodevelopment and the impact of life experience on neural structure and function (Teicher et al. 2016, Shonkoff et al. 2014, Perry et al. 1995), interpersonal neurobiology (Siegel 2001, Cozolino 2010) and emotion focussed (Greenberg 2010) and sensorimotor therapies (Fisher 2011, Ogden, Minton, and Pain 2006). The concept of attachment has also become central to understanding the dynamics of threat and safety in romantic relationships (Mikulincer and Shaver 2007, Johnson 2011). These fields of research have changed practice – from infant mental health to couple therapy – they are important for the whole of Humpty's life experience.

The attachment literature is replete with both neurobiological and relational research that confirms the impact of *sense of safety* on mental and physical well-being. An attachment relationship is described as a 'safety regulating system' (Allen and Manning 2007, 23) comprising differing caregiving and care-receiving systems. Early childhood experiences of safety facilitate affect regulation, neural networks and connectivity, integration of sensory and narrative information, language capacity and the formation of a stable sense of self (Schore 2003, Mikulincer 1995, Schore 2001, Lupien et al. 2009, Shonkoff et al. 2014, Shonkoff et al. 2012, Teicher et al. 2016). These early experiences affect adult cortical capacity to down-regulate emotion, self-soothe, establish a stable sense of self and co-regulate trust in intimate relationships. The impact at a neurological level influences lifetime mental and physical health (Schore 2001, 1996, Njiokiktjien and Verschoor 2012). As summarised by Bessel van der Kolk: 'If you feel safe and loved, your brain becomes specialised in exploration, play and cooperation. If you are frightened and unwanted, it specialises in managing feelings of fear and abandonment' (Van Der Kolk 2014a, 56).

Sense of safety: An essential aspect of therapeutic relationship

Sense of safety is a way to describe a goal of therapeutic interaction in any setting. It could therefore be used to help practitioners engage with patients, employees, students and colleagues. It could be an overarching goal of the process, as well as the content of constructive interactions.

Sense of safety impacts our capacity to connect to others: 'when features of safety are detected, autonomic reactions promote open receptivity with others, but when features of threat are detected autonomic reactions promote a closed state limiting the awareness of others' (Geller and Porges 2014, 183). In the literature on therapeutic relationships, safety is noted to increase trust, warmth and disclosure (Romano, Fitzpatrick, and Janzen 2008) and is described as a physiological state in both clinician and patient that creates 'optimal conditions for growth and change' (Geller and Porges 2014, 178). In the primary care setting, this is known as 'abiding' (Scott et al. 2008) or 'shared presence' (Ventres and Frankel 2015). Shared presence includes reflecting on self and other, accepting diversity of perspectives and expectations, seeing the patient through showing interest, sensing feelings, listening to story, touching with sensitivity and using time wisely (Ventres and Frankel 2015). Somatosensory forms of therapy harness this capacity for safety, soothing from both 'top down' (brain to body) and 'bottom up' (body to brain) (Chiesa, Serretti, and Jakobsen 2013). Shari Geller and Stephen Porges affirm the importance of a calm therapist facilitating the 'neuroception of safety' (Geller and Porges 2014, 189) with 'warmth and prosody of voice, soft eye contact, open body posture, and receptive and accepting stance' (Geller and Porges 2014, 184). They also declare that 'client safety ... [is] a core prerequisite for effective therapeutic work regardless of the therapeutic approach' (Geller and Porges 2014, 188).

Attachment theory is already used by consultant liaison psychiatrists who focus their care on increasing 'felt security' of their distressed inpatients (Maunder and Hunter 2016, 10). The trauma-informed clinical process of maintaining a 'therapeutic window' (Briere 2002) makes the clinical encounter safe enough so that the person can 'feel without resorting to defences' (Courtois 2004, 421). The current trauma-informed guidelines reinforce that priority: 'facilitate patient safety at all times' (Kezelman and Stavropoulos 2019, 34) based on Christine Courtois' assertion that the 'first order of treatment is to establish conditions of safety to the fullest extent possible' (Courtois and Ford 2009, 91).

Sense of safety: A physiological reality

Reviews of transdisciplinary research confirm the impact of threatening life experience on the whole person. Individual appraisal of internal or external threat impacts the hypothalamic-pituitary-adrenal (HPA) axis, sympathetic-adrenal-medullary (SAM) axis and endocrine, immune, neurological and metabolic systems (Lynch and Kirkengen 2019). Neuropsychology research confirms the preverbal, sensory, memorial and neurological encoding of threat (Cozolino 2010) in response to fear-inducing or conditioning memories (Phillips and LeDoux 1992). Threat can impact the interaction of the active sympathetic and recuperative parasympathetic autonomic systems – as Pat Ogden reminds, the unmodulated sympathetic system can remain 'primed for threat and reacting to danger long since over' (Ogden, Minton, and Pain 2006, 21). At a cellular level, glucocorticoid regulation is impacted by stress leading to oxidative stress, inflammation, cellular apoptosis and telomere shortening, and epigenetic changes (Shaughnessy et al. 2014, Picard, Juster, and McEwen 2014). Researchers into multimorbidity (Tomasdottir et al. 2015) and depression (Roy and Campbell 2013) acknowledge the potential common pathway between stress, even existential unease (Tomasdottir et al. 2016), and physiology.

Modern-day stress research, as per Selye's original observations, describes stress as a 'non-specific response' to alarm (Van Praag, de Kloet, and van Os 2004, 12) that only occurs if the perceived stressor is more than the individual can adapt to (Van Praag, de Kloet, and van Os 2004, 13). Selye coined the term 'stress' to name the impact on the organism of what he termed a 'stressor', which can be conceptualised as threats to *sense of safety*. He crossed disciplinary boundaries to suggest a unifying concept – called the General Adaptation Syndrome – that named the loss of capacity of all organisms to adapt to stressors as 'diseases of adaptation' (Selye 1950, 1956). This concept is a foundation for recent research into allostatic load, multimorbidity and chronic disease (Tomasdottir et al. 2015, England-Mason et al. 2018, Delpierre et al. 2016, McEwen 2000, Lupien et al. 2009).

Stress, beyond normal challenge, is defined as 'tolerable' or 'toxic' stress based on the presence or absence of 'the buffering protection of a supportive adult relationship' (Shonkoff et al. 2012, e236). Fear modulation, through relationship, is a significant 'hidden regulator' of physiological health (Coan, Schaefer, and Davidson 2006, 1038). The extensive attachment, social stress, social rejection and loneliness literature documents the impact of both adult and childhood relationships on physiology. From wound healing and neurological pain sensitivity to cardiac death rates, inflammation, endocrine dysregulation and synaptic connectivity, experiencing relational safety impacts health (Uchino, Cacioppo, and Kiecolt-Glaser 1996, Eisenberger et al. 2011, Slavich et al. 2010, Kosfeld et al. 2005, Bartz et al. 2010, Kirsch et al. 2005, Hammock and Young 2006, Conway et al. 2018, Valtorta et al. 2016, Gouin et al. 2010, Uchino et al. 2018, Perry et al. 1995).

When threat is chronic or unbuffered by relationships perceived as supportive, the capacity of the organism to adapt to stress (termed 'allostasis') (McEwen and Wingfield 2003) can become overwhelmed. The resulting allostatic overload causes multisystem physiological dysregulation (Wiley et al. 2016) and increased morbidity and mortality (Juster et al. 2011, Juster, McEwen, and Lupien 2010). Those who research the impact of allostatic overload on the body describe the impact of psychosocial and physical threat (Fleshner and Laudenslager 2004) on host defence mechanisms. This alters the interconnected immune, endocrine, metabolic and neurologic systems (McEwen and Wingfield 2003, McEwen 2007, Van Praag, de Kloet, and van Os 2004). Robert-Paul Juster and colleagues (2016, 1117) describe this as 'equifinality and multifinality in stress phenomena'. Allostatic load impacts the whole person, including genetic telomeres, cellular senescence, organ function and longevity (Picard, Juster, and McEwen 2014). Psychoneuroimmunology, another transdisciplinary field, researches the impact of threat on the immune system and endocrine systems, including pro-inflammatory cytokines (Fagundes, Glaser, and Kiecolt-Glaser 2013, Dickerson et al. 2009).

Early life stress has been named as an 'unrecognised confound in psychiatric neuroimaging studies that calls into question the interpretation of prior results' (Teicher and Samson 2016, 623). Early life social stressors have been identified as underlying 'transdiagnostic, and not disorder specific, liabilities to psychopathology' (Conway et al. 2018). Overwhelm has also been linked to physiological addictive processes (Volkow et al. 2010). The large epidemiological Adverse Childhood Experiences (ACE) study prospectively followed up survivors of adverse childhood experiences, confirming a direct dose-dependent (more adversity=more impact) link between early childhood experiences and morbidity and mortality (Felitti et al. 1998). Long-term physiological and neurodevelopmental health impacts of adverse childhood experiences have been established by the ACE (Dube et al. 2003) and Maltreatment and Abuse Chronology of Exposure (MACE) (Teicher and Parigger 2015) studies. The timing, type and intensity of these experiences is also relevant (Schalinski et al. 2016) with distinct developmental patterns (Teicher and Parigger 2015). These key adverse childhood experiences of invasion, disconnection and confusion (see Chapter Five) are outlined in Table 4.1. These studies are so conclusive that they define a bare minimum of

Table 4.1 Adverse Childhood Experiences with Proven Physiological Impacts

Adverse Childhood Experiences with proven physiological impacts

Disconnection	Invasion	'Missing' parent
Physical neglect	Physical abuse	Absent parent
Emotional neglect	Sexual abuse	Intoxicated parent
Non-verbal emotional abuse*	Witnessing interparental violence	Hospitalised parent
Emotional abuse	Witnessing violence against siblings*	Incarcerated parent
	Peer physical bullying*	

Source: *Collated using information from Felitti (1998) and Teicher (2015) [marked with*]*

life experiences that are relevant to the assessment of distress. For the generalist, these experiences also represent early intervention opportunities that are relevant to the health of our communities.

Sense of safety: **Attending to a *gestalt* experience**

Linn Getz (1999), an experienced GP, raises a question relevant to this discussion of threat, safety and coping:

> Beyond treatment resistant somatic symptoms, unexplainable autonomic or neurological experiences or destructive personality traits, there may be a 'gestalt' which we never learned to recognise in medical school. The gestalt reflects the fact that at one time in life this person was overwhelmed. Human integrity was violated and last resort coping strategies were activated.
>
> (Getz 1999, 68)

A stakeholder echoed this awareness saying:

> What if most of what traditionally is called 'psychopathology' actually is a consequence of threatening experiences/threat to life, existence or personal integrity. If so, the original loss of safety due to real threat can only be healed by a person's regained trust in being safe. (gp-a)

This aligns with Maslow's previously mentioned and influential concept of safety as a meta-need (Maslow 1954, 8). He identified and named human needs in a way that continues to have relevance and authenticity, including needs for physiological homeostasis, safety, belonging and love, esteem, and self-actualisation. Although the hierarchy and the lack of laboratory confirmation of his theory have been critiqued (Geller 1982, Neher 1991, Trigg 2004), his theory attempted to counter the impact of behaviourism (only observing the person from outside as an object of study) and the atomisation of medical care – the 'body parts approach' (Hunter 1999). Maslow saw the experience of safety as crossing cultural barriers – as a fundamental need of the whole person.

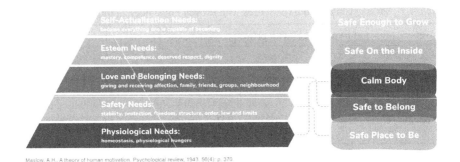

Maslow, A.H., A theory of human motivation. Psychological review, 1943. 50(4): p. 370

Figure 4.2 Reframing Maslow: *sense of safety whole person goals.*

Maslow sought to see the whole. In fact he wrote: 'Perhaps what we speak of as separate disease entities in the medical model are actually superficial and idiosyncratic reactions to a deeper general illness' (Maslow 1954, 80). The concept of *sense of safety* integrates all the layers of Maslow's hierarchy of needs and sees them as interdependent rather than a hierarchy. All the elements of his hierarchy outlined in Figure 4.2 are seen as contributors towards whole person *sense of safety*. For example, physiological homeostasis (Calm Body), safety (Safe Place to Be), love and belonging (Safe to Belong), self-esteem (Safe on the Inside) and self-actualisation (Safe Enough to Grow). The *sense of safety* concept does not see these needs as hierarchical but as linked in complex feedback loops requiring *sense of safety* across the whole person. As depicted in Figure 4.2, these healing-oriented *sense of safety whole person goals* place the physiological experience of 'calm body' centrally. This reflects the physical embodied person impacting and being impacted externally by context (Safe Place to Be) and relationships (Safe to Belong) and internally by inner experiences (Safe on the Inside) and meaning (Safe Enough to Grow).

Appraising *sense of safety* and *loss of sense of safety* may offer a way to notice this *gestalt*. Noticing anything – past or present, internal or external, conscious or unconscious, accurately or inaccurately perceived – that has ever caused overwhelm. These goals intentionally draw attention towards healing of the whole person.

Sense of safety could be seen as a simplistic solution to a complex problem, a shared language that is too limited to be useful. It is counter-intuitive that such an ordinary phrase could integrate complex dynamic aspects of the person in distress – even though it originates from a word that means 'whole' (Nilsen et al. 2004). And yet, clinicians who were consulted about this idea could see that its simplicity was also one of its strengths. An academic psychiatrist with expertise in attachment responded to the *sense of safety* concept:

> Overall, I think the greatest strength of the approach you are describing in the simplest idea at its core – that people in primary care are often bothered by distress that emerges from their lives in all of their complexity and that this can be

missed or misconstrued by conventional approaches to the physician-patient interaction ... the approach you are developing has great potential. (mhc-a)

When assessed over multiple domains, including unconscious or unnoticed perceptions, and in reflective dialogue between clinician and patient, *sense of safety* has the potential to give a clear snapshot of a person's whole experience and to increase the person's capacity to be aware of and improve their relative *sense of safety*.

In this book, I propose the concept of *sense of safety* as a coherent way to approach people who are distressed. This concept, although on first glance a simplistic and idealistic approach to the person, is grounded in clinical reality, philosophical legitimacy, new cross-disciplinary (or transdisciplinary) science and stakeholder and academic consultation. It has been developed by a generalist clinician in response to very real scientific and humane concerns about the status quo that fragments the person in order to treat disease (in the health setting) or behaviour (in the school or office) while often ignoring the wellbeing of that same person. This concept of *sense of safety*, as will be explored in later chapters, includes not just a sense of comfort but also a sense of capacity or courage to engage with life or grow. It is also designed to include the voice of the distressed in their sense of their own wellbeing and be applicable to all people – including those who care for the distressed in their worlds.

Note

1 "Disenfranchised grief" is a term coined by Ken Doka to describe grief that the sufferer often has to suffer alone as their community does not recognise it (e.g., death of a pet who was more like a child, death of a secret lover, death from something shameful).

References

2019. 'Hygge.' Accessed 22/5/2020. https://en.wikipedia.org/wiki/Hygge.

Allen, J.G. 2013. *Restoring mentalizing in attachment relationships: Treating trauma with plain old therapy*. Washington: American Psychiatric Publishing.

Allen, Joseph P., and Nell Manning. 2007. 'From safety to affect regulation: Attachment from the vantage point of adolescence.' *New Directions for Child and Adolescent Development*. (117):23–39. doi:10.1002/cd.192.

Bartz, Jennifer A., Jamil Zaki, Niall Bolger, Eric Hollander, Natasha N. Ludwig, Alexander Kolevzon, and Kevin N. Ochsner. 2010. 'Oxytocin selectively improves empathic accuracy.' *Psychological Science* 21 (10):1426–1428.

Blatz, W.E. 1973. 'The theory of human security.' In *Child development: Selected readings*, edited by L.M. Brockman, J.H. Whiteley, and J.P. Zubek, 150–166. Toronto: McClelland and Stewart Ltd.

Bowlby, John. 1979. 'The Bowlby-Ainsworth attachment theory.' *Behavioral and Brain Sciences* 2 (4):637–638.

Briere, John, ed. 2002. *Treating adult survivors of severe childhood*. Edited by J.E.B. Myers, L. Berliner, J. Briere, C.T. Hendrix, C. Jenny and T.A. Reid, *The APSAC handbook on child maltreatment*, 175–203. Thousand Oaks, CA: Sage Publications, Inc.

Calhoun, L.G., and R.G. Tedeschi, eds. 2006. *Handbook of posttraumatic growth. Research and practice*. Mahwah, NJ: Lawrence Erlbaum Associates.

Carleton, R. Nicholas. 2016a. 'Fear of the unknown: One fear to rule them all?' *Journal of Anxiety Disorders* 41:5–21.

Carleton, R. Nicholas. 2016b. 'Into the unknown: A review and synthesis of contemporary models involving uncertainty.' *Journal of Anxiety Disorders* 39:30–43.

Carmeli, Abraham, Daphna Brueller, and Jane E. Dutton. 2009. 'Learning behaviours in the workplace: The role of high-quality interpersonal relationships and psychological safety.' *Systems Research and Behavioral Science: The Official Journal of the International Federation for Systems Research* 26 (1):81–98.

Chiesa, Alberto, Alessandro Serretti, and Janus Christian Jakobsen. 2013. 'Mindfulness: Top-down or bottom-up emotion regulation strategy?' *Clinical Psychology Review* 33 (1):82–96.

Christakis, Nicholas A., and Theodore J. Iwashyna. 2003. 'The health impact of health care on families: A matched cohort study of hospice use by decedents and mortality outcomes in surviving, widowed spouses.' *Social Science & Medicine* 57 (3):465–475.

Coan, James A., Hillary S. Schaefer, and Richard J. Davidson. 2006. 'Lending a hand social regulation of the neural response to threat.' *Psychological Science* 17 (12):1032–1039.

Conway, Christopher C., Elizabeth B. Raposa, Constance Hammen, and Patricia A. Brennan. 2018. 'Transdiagnostic pathways from early social stress to psychopathology: A 20-year prospective study.' *Journal of Child Psychology and Psychiatry* 59 (8):855–862.

Courtois, C.A. 2004. 'Complex trauma, complex reactions: Assessment and treatment.' *Psychotherapy: Theory, Research, Practice, Training* 41 (4):412–425.

Courtois, C.A., and Julian Ford, eds. 2009. *Treating complex traumatic stress. An evidence based guide*. New York: The Guilford Press.

Cozolino, Louis. 2010. *The Neuroscience of psychotherapy: Healing the social brain (Norton Series on Interpersonal Neurobiology)*. New York: WW Norton & Company.

Delpierre, Cyrille, Cristina Barboza-Solis, Jerome Torrisani, Muriel Darnaudery, Melanie Bartley, David Blane, Michelle Kelly-Irving, Linn Getz, Margret Olafia Tomasdottir, and Tony Robertson. 2016. 'Origins of health inequalities: The case for Allostatic Load.' *Longitudinal and Life Course Studies* 7 (1):79–103.

Dickerson, Sally S., Shelly L. Gable, Michael R. Irwin, Najib Aziz, and Margaret E. Kemeny. 2009. 'Social-evaluative threat and proinflammatory cytokine regulation: An experimental laboratory investigation.' *Psychological Science* 20 (10):1237–1244.

Dube, Shanta R., Vincent J. Felitti, Maxia Dong, Wayne H. Giles, and Robert F. Anda. 2003. 'The impact of adverse childhood experiences on health problems: Evidence from four birth cohorts dating back to 1900.' *Preventive Medicine* 37 (3):268–277.

Edmondson, Amy. 2004. 'Psychological safety, trust and learning in organisation: A group-level lens.' In *Trust and distrust in organisations: Dilemmas and approaches*, edited by R.M. Kramer, and K.S. Cook, 239–272. New York: Russell Sage Foundation.

Eisenberger, N.I., S.L. Master, and T.K. Inagaki. 2011. 'Attachment figures activate a safety signal-related neural region and reduce pain experience.' *Proceedings of the National Academy of Sciences* 108 (28):11721–11726.

England-Mason, Gillian, Rebecca Casey, Mark Ferro, Harriet L. MacMillan, Lil Tonmyr, and Andrea Gonzalez. 2018. 'Child maltreatment and adult multimorbidity: Results from the Canadian community health survey.' *Canadian Journal of Public Health* 109:561–572. https://doi.org/10.17269/s41997-018-0069-y.

Enns, Carolyn Zerbe, Jean Campbell, Christine A. Courtois, Michael C. Gottlieb, Karen P. Lese, Mary S. Gilbert, and Linda Forrest. 1998. 'Working with adult clients who may have experienced childhood abuse: Recommendations for assessment and practice.' *Professional Psychology: Research and Practice* 29 (3):245–256.

Fagundes, Christopher P., Ronald Glaser, and Janice K. Kiecolt-Glaser. 2013. 'Stressful early life experiences and immune dysregulation across the lifespan.' *Brain, Behavior, and Immunity* 27:8–12.

Felitti, V.J., R.F. Anda, D. Nordenberg, D.F. Williamson, A.M. Spitz, V. Edwards, M.P. Koss, and J.S. Marks. 1998. 'Relationship of childhood abuse and household dysfunction to many of the leading causes of death in adults: The Adverse Childhood Experiences (ACE) study.' *American Journal of Preventive Medicine* 14 (4):245–258.

Fisher, Janina. 2011. 'Sensorimotor approaches to trauma treatment.' *Advances in Psychiatric Treatment* 17 (3):171–177.

Fleshner, Monika, and Mark L. Laudenslager. 2004. 'Psychoneuroimmunology: Then and now.' *Behavioral and Cognitive Neuroscience Reviews* 3 (2):114–130.

Frewen, Paul, Kathy Hegadoren, Nick J. Coupland, Brian H. Rowe, Richard W.J. Neufeld, and Ruth Lanius. 2015. 'Trauma related altered states of consciousness (TRASC) and functional impairment 1: Prospective study in acutely traumatized persons.' *Journal of Trauma & Dissociation* 16 (5):500–519. doi:10.1080/15299732.2015.1022925.

Geller, Leonard. 1982. 'The failure of self-actualization theory: A critique of Carl Rogers and Abraham Maslow.' *Journal of Humanistic Psychology* 22 (2):56–73.

Geller, Shari M., and Stephen W. Porges. 2014. 'Therapeutic presence: Neurophysiological mechanisms mediating feeling safe in therapeutic relationships.' *Journal of Psychotherapy Integration* 24 (3):178–192.

Getz, Linn. 1999. '"Unexplainable" medical histories and childhood sexual abuse: New doctoral thesis tells you how to investigate the links.' *Scandinavian Journal of Primary Health Care* 17 (2):68–71.

Gouin, Jean-Philippe, C. Sue Carter, Hossein Pournajafi-Nazarloo, Ronald Glaser, William B. Malarkey, Timothy J. Loving, Jeffrey Stowell, and Janice K. Kiecolt-Glaser. 2010. 'Marital behavior, oxytocin, vasopressin, and wound healing.' *Psychoneuroendocrinology* 35 (7):1082–1090.

Greenberg, Leslie S. 2010. 'Emotion-focused therapy: A clinical synthesis.' *Focus* 8 (1):32–42.

Hammock, Elizabeth A.D., and Larry J. Young. 2006. 'Oxytocin, vasopressin and pair bonding: Implications for autism.' *Philosophical Transactions of the Royal Society of London B: Biological Sciences* 361 (1476):2187–2198.

Herman, Judith L. 2015. *Trauma and recovery: The aftermath of violence – from domestic abuse to political terror.* Hachette UK.

Horowitz, Mardi J., Bryna Siegel, Are Holen, George A. Bonanno, Constance Milbrath, and Charles H. Stinson. 2003. 'Diagnostic criteria for complicated grief disorder.' *Focus* 1 (3):290–298.

Hunter, Puggy (Arnold). 1999. 'Searching for a new way of thinking in aboriginal health.' *NACCHO News* 3 (July):1–2.

Janoff-Bulman, Ronnie. 1985. 'The aftermath of victimization: Rebuilding shattered assumptions.' *Trauma and its Wake* 1:15–35.

Johnson, Sue. 2011. *Hold me tight: Your guide to the most successful approach to building loving relationships.* Hachette UK.

Juster, Robert-Paul, Gustav Bizik, Martin Picard, Genevieve Arsenault-Lapierre, Shireen Sindi, Lyane Trepanier, Marie-France Marin, Nathalie Wan, Zoran Sekerovic, and Catherine Lord. 2011. 'A transdisciplinary perspective of chronic stress in relation to psychopathology throughout life span development.' *Development and Psychopathology* 23 (3):725–776.

Juster, Robert-Paul, Bruce S. McEwen, and Sonia J. Lupien. 2010. 'Allostatic load biomarkers of chronic stress and impact on health and cognition.' *Neuroscience & Biobehavioral Reviews* 35 (1):2–16.

Juster, Robert-Paul, Jennifer J. Russell, Daniel Almeida, and Martin Picard. 2016. 'Allostatic load and comorbidities: A mitochondrial, epigenetic, and evolutionary perspective.' *Development and Psychopathology* 28 (4pt1):1117–1146.

Kerns, Kathryn A., Brittany L. Mathews, Amanda J. Koehn, Cierra T. Williams, and Shannon Siener-Ciesla. 2015. 'Assessing both safe haven and secure base support in parent–child relationships.' *Attachment & Human Development* 17 (4):337–353.

Kezelman, Cathy, and Pam Stavropoulos. 2012. *'The Last Frontier': Practice guidelines for treatment of complex Trauma and Trauma informed care and service delivery.* Sydney: Adults Surviving Child Abuse.

Kezelman, Cathy, and Pam Stavropoulos. 2019. *Practice guidelines for treatment of complex Trauma.* Sydney: Blue Knot Foundation

Kirsch, Peter, Christine Esslinger, Qiang Chen, Daniela Mier, Stefanie Lis, Sarina Siddhanti, Harald Gruppe, Venkata S. Mattay, Bernd Gallhofer, and Andreas Meyer-Lindenberg. 2005. 'Oxytocin modulates neural circuitry for social cognition and fear in humans.' *Journal of Neuroscience* 25 (49):11489–11493.

Kosfeld, Michael, Markus Heinrichs, Paul J. Zak, Urs Fischbacher, and Ernst Fehr. 2005. 'Oxytocin increases trust in humans.' *Nature* 435 (7042):673.

Kuo, Frances E., Magdalena Bacaicoa, and William C. Sullivan. 1998. 'Transforming inner-city landscapes trees, sense of safety, and preference.' *Environment and Behavior* 30 (1):28–59.

Lupien, Sonia J., Bruce S. McEwen, Megan R. Gunnar, and Christine Heim. 2009. 'Effects of stress throughout the lifespan on the brain, behaviour and cognition.' *Nature Reviews Neuroscience* 10 (6):434–445.

Lynch, J.M., and A.L. Kirkengen. 2019. 'Biology and experience intertwined: Trauma, neglect and physical health.' In *Humanising mental health care in Australia: A guide to Trauma-informed approaches*, edited by R. Benjamin, J. Haliburn, and S. King, 195–207. Sydney: CRC Press Taylor and Francis Group, Routledge.

Maslow, A.H. 1954. *Motivation and personality third edition.* Edited by R. Frager, J. Fadiman, C. McReynolds, and R. Cox. New York: Harper Collins Publishers.

Maunder, Robert G., and Jonathan J. Hunter. 2001. 'Attachment and psychosomatic medicine: Developmental contributions to stress and disease.' 63 (4):556–567.

Maunder, Robert G., and Jonathan J. Hunter. 2016. 'Can patients be "attached" to healthcare providers? An observational study to measure attachment phenomena in patient–provider relationships.' *BMJ Open* 6 (5):e011068. doi:10.1136/bmjopen-2016-011068.

McEwen, Bruce S. 2000. 'Allostasis and allostatic load: Implications for neuropsychopharmacology.' *Neuropsychopharmacology* 22 (2):108–124.

McEwen, Bruce S. 2007. 'Physiology and neurobiology of stress and adaptation: Central role of the brain.' *Physiological Reviews* 87 (3):873–904.

McEwen, Bruce S., and John C. Wingfield. 2003. 'The concept of allostasis in biology and biomedicine.' *Hormones and Behavior* 43 (1):2–15.

Mikulincer, Mario 1995. 'Attachment style and the mental representation of the self.' *Journal of Personality and Social Psychology* 69 (6):1203–1215.

Mikulincer, Mario, and Phillip R. Shaver. 2007. *Attachment in adulthood: Structure, dynamics, and change.* New York: Guilford Press.

Milberg, Anna, Maria Friedrichsen, Maria Jakobsson, Eva-Carin Nilsson, Birgitta Niskala, Maria Olsson, Rakel Wåhlberg, and Barbro Krevers. 2014. 'Patients' sense of security during palliative care – what are the influencing factors?' *Journal of Pain and Symptom Management* 48 (1):45–55.

Murthy, Vivek Hallegere. 2020. *Together: The healing power of human connection in a sometimes lonely world.* New York, NY: Harper Collins Publishers.

Neher, Andrew. 1991. 'Maslow's theory of motivation: A critique.' *Journal of Humanistic Psychology* 31 (3):89–112.

Nilsen, Per, D.S. Hudson, Agneta Kullberg, Toomas Timpka, Robert Ekman, and Kent Lindqvist. 2004. 'Making sense of safety.' *Injury Prevention* 10 (2):71–73.

Njiokiktjien, Charles, and Catharina Anna Verschoor. 2012. 'The role of the hippocampus in neural mechanisms of attachment and attachment disorders: A review.' In *Brain Lesion localization and developmental functions,* edited by D. Riva, Charles Njiokiktjien, and S. Bulgheroni, 157–172. Montrouge: John Libbey Eurotext.

Ogden, P., K. Minton, and C Pain, eds. 2006. *Trauma and the body. A sensorimotor approach to psychotherapy.* New York: W.W. Norton and Company Inc.

Perry, Bruce D., Ronnie A. Pollard, Toi L. Blakley, William L. Baker, and Domenico Vigilante. 1995. 'Childhood trauma, the neurobiology of adaptation, and use dependent development of the brain: How states become traits.' *Infant Mental Health Journal* 16 (4):271–291.

Phillips, R.G., and J.E. LeDoux. 1992. 'Differential contribution of amygdala and hippocampus to cued and contextual fear conditioning.' *Behavioral Neuroscience* 106 (2):274–285.

Picard, Martin, Robert-Paul Juster, and Bruce S. McEwen. 2014. 'Mitochondrial allostatic load puts the "gluc" back in glucocorticoids.' *Nature Reviews Endocrinology* 10 (5):303–310.

Porges, S. 2014. *Connectedness as a biological imperative.* Australian Childhood Foundation Conference, Melbourne.

Powell, Bert, Glen Cooper, Kent Hoffman, and Bob Marvin. 2013. *The circle of security intervention: Enhancing attachment in early parent-child relationships.* New York, NY: Guilford Publications.

Rappoport, Alan. 1997. 'The patient's search for safety: The organizing principle in psychotherapy.' *Psychotherapy: Theory, Research, Practice, Training* 34 (3):250–261.

Romano, Vera, Marilyn Fitzpatrick, and Jennifer Janzen. 2008. 'The secure-base hypothesis: Global attachment, attachment to counselor, and session exploration in psychotherapy.' *Journal of Counseling Psychology* 55 (4):495–504.

Ross, Colin A. 2000. *The trauma model: A solution to the problem of comorbidity in psychiatry.* Richardson, TX: Manitou Communications.

Roy, Amrita, and M. Karen Campbell. 2013. 'A unifying framework for depression: Bridging the major biological and psychosocial theories through stress.' *Clinical & Investigative Medicine* 36 (4):170–190.

Rutter, Michael. 1995. 'Clinical implications of attachment concepts: Retrospect and prospect.' *Journal of Child Psychology and Psychiatry* 36 (4):549–571.

Schalinski, Inga, Martin H. Teicher, Daniel Nischk, Eva Hinderer, Oliver Müller, and Brigitte Rockstroh. 2016. 'Type and timing of adverse childhood experiences differentially affect severity of PTSD, dissociative and depressive symptoms in adult inpatients.' *BMC Psychiatry* 16 (1):295. doi:10.1186/s12888-016-1004-5.

Schore, A.N. 1996. 'The experience-dependent maturation of a regulatory system in the orbital prefrontal cortex and the origin of developmental psychopathology.' *Development and Psychopathology* 8:59–88.

Schore, A.N. 2001. 'Effects of a secure attachment relationship on right brain development, affect regulation, and infant mental health.' *Infant Mental Health Journal* 22 (1–2):7–66.

Schore, A.N. 2003. *Affect regulation & disorders of the self, series on interpersonal neurobiology.* New York: WW Norton & Company.

Scott, J.G, D. Cohen, B. DiCicco Bloom, W. Miller, K. Stange, and B. Crabtree. 2008. 'Understanding healing relationships in primary care.' *Annals of Family Medicine* 6 (4):315–322.

Selye, Hans. 1950. 'Stress and the general adaptation syndrome.' *British Medical Journal* 4667:1383–1392.

Selye, Hans. 1956. *The stress of life.* New York: McGraw Hill Book Company.

Shaughnessy, Daniel T., Kimberly McAllister, Leroy Worth, Astrid C. Haugen, Joel N. Meyer, Frederick E. Domann, Bennett Van Houten, Raul Mostoslavsky, Scott J. Bultman, and Andrea A. Baccarelli. 2014. 'Mitochondria, energetics, epigenetics, and cellular responses to stress.' *Environmental Health Perspectives (Online)* 122 (12):1271.

Shonkoff, Jack P., Andrew S. Garner, Benjamin S. Siegel, Mary I. Dobbins, Marian F. Earls, Laura McGuinn, John Pascoe, David L. Wood, Committee on Psychosocial Aspects of Child, Family Health, Adoption Committee on Early Childhood, and Dependent Care. 2012. 'The lifelong effects of early childhood adversity and toxic stress.' *Pediatrics* 129 (1):e232–e246.

Shonkoff, Jack P., W.T. Boyce, J. Cameron, G.J. Duncan, N.A. Fox, M.R. Gunnar, and R.A. Thompson. 2014. *Excessive stress disrupts the architecture of the developing brain.* In Working Paper 3 Updated edition. Centre on the Developing Child, Harvard University: National Scientific Council on the Developing Child.

Siegel, D.J. 2001. 'Toward an interpersonal neurobiology of the developing mind: Attachment relationships, "mindsight," and neural integration.' *Infant Mental Health Journal* 22 (1–2):67–94.

Slavich, George M., Baldwin M. Way, Naomi I. Eisenberger, and Shelley E. Taylor. 2010. 'Neural sensitivity to social rejection is associated with inflammatory responses to social stress.' *Proceedings of the National Academy of Sciences* 107 (33):14817–14822.

Svenaeus, Fredrik. 2001. 'The phenomenology of health and illness.' In *Handbook of phenomenology and medicine*, edited by Kay Toombs, 87–108. Dordrecht, Netherlands: Kluwer Academic.

Teicher, Martin H., and Angelika Parigger. 2015. 'The "Maltreatment and Abuse Chronology of Exposure (MACE)" scale for the retrospective assessment of abuse and neglect during development.' *PLOS ONE* 10 (2):e0117423. https://doi.org/10.1371/j ournal.pone.0117423.

Teicher, Martin H., and Jacqueline A. Samson. 2016. 'Annual research review: Enduring neurobiological effects of childhood abuse and neglect.' *Journal of Child Psychology and Psychiatry* 57 (3):241–266.

Teicher, Martin H., Jacqueline A. Samson, Carl M. Anderson, and Kyoko Ohashi. 2016. 'The effects of childhood maltreatment on brain structure, function and connectivity.' *Nature Reviews Neuroscience* 17 (10):652–666.

Tomasdottir, Margret Olafia, Johann Agust Sigurdsson, Halfdan Petursson, Anna Luise Kirkengen, Steinar Krokstad, Bruce McEwen, Irene Hetlevik, and Linn Getz. 2015. 'Self reported childhood difficulties, adult multimorbidity and allostatic load. A cross-sectional analysis of the Norwegian HUNT study.' *PLOS ONE* 10 (6):e0130591. https://doi.org/10.1371/journal.pone.0130591.

Tomasdottir, Margret Olafia, Johann Agust Sigurdsson, Halfdan Petursson, Anna Luise Kirkengen, Tom Ivar Lund Nilsen, Irene Hetlevik, and Linn Getz. 2016. 'Does "existential unease" predict adult multimorbidity? Analytical cohort study on embodiment based on the Norwegian HUNT population.' *BMJ Open* 6 (11):e012602. doi:10.1136/bmjopen-2016-012602.

Trigg, Andrew B. 2004. 'Deriving the Engel curve: Pierre Bourdieu and the social critique of Maslow's hierarchy of needs.' *Review of Social Economy* 62 (3):393–406.

Uchino, Bert N., John T. Cacioppo, and Janice K. Kiecolt-Glaser. 1996. 'The relationship between social support and physiological processes: A review with emphasis on underlying mechanisms and implications for health.' *Psychological bulletin* 119 (3):488–531.

Uchino, Bert N., Ryan Trettevik, Robert G. Kent de Grey, Sierra Cronan, Jasara Hogan, and Brian R.W. Baucom. 2018. 'Social support, social integration, and inflammatory cytokines: A meta-analysis.' *Health Psychology* 37 (5):462–471.

Valtorta, Nicole K., Mona Kanaan, Simon Gilbody, Sara Ronzi, and Barbara Hanratty. 2016. 'Loneliness and social isolation as risk factors for coronary heart disease and stroke: Systematic review and meta-analysis of longitudinal observational studies.' *Heart* 102 (13):1009–1016.

Van Der Kolk, Bessel. 2014a. *The body keeps the score*. New York: Viking.

Van Der Kolk, Bessel. 2014b. *The body keeps the score: Mind, brain, body in the transformation of Trauma*. New York: Viking.

Van Praag, Herman M., E. Ron de Kloet, and Jim van Os. 2004. *Stress, the brain and depression*. Cambridge: Cambridge University Press.

Ventres, William B., and Richard M. Frankel. 2015. 'Shared presence in physician-patient communication: A graphic representation.' *Families, Systems, & Health* 33 (3):270–279. http://doi.org/10.1037/fsh0000123.

Volkow, Nora D, Gene-Jack Wang, Joanna S Fowler, Dardo Tomasi, Frank Telang, and Ruben Baler. 2010. 'Addiction: Decreased reward sensitivity and increased expectation sensitivity conspire to overwhelm the brain's control circuit.' *Bioessays* 32 (9):748–755.

Wiley, Joshua F., Tara L. Gruenewald, Arun S. Karlamangla, and Teresa E. Seeman. 2016. 'Modeling multisystem physiological dysregulation.' *Psychosomatic Medicine* 78 (3):290–301.

5 Senses matter: Senses protect integrity, connection and coherence

- What Humpty senses matters
- Sensing and sense-making are interconnected ways to understand the world
- Sensing is a form of communication across the whole person from the cellular to the communal
- Sensing has a purpose of protecting integrity, connection and coherence

As discussed in previous chapters, Humpty is a whole made of many parts. When Humpty is well, he does not experience himself in parts. If Humpty is out on a bush walk, he can notice the birds, the crunch of the forest floor, the smells, the weight of his backpack. He can enjoy the conversation and company of people he is with, as well as imagine the view he is going to see. He is able to be concurrently aware of all of these aspects of his experience. Noticing his inner experience, Humpty is able to take in inputs from various sources at once to help him to organise himself, help him to appraise his situation and help him to perceive his capacity to cope and make his way in the world. His interconnected system takes in his environment and links it to his inner and bodily experience, and 'makes sense' of what is going on.

If, however, a snake appeared on the path ahead, Humpty's capacity to sense becomes narrowed, prioritising attention towards what is important and losing awareness of the wider view. If the snake is a few metres away, Humpty experiences alarm that narrows his attention and his body prepares for fight or flight. His eardrum shifts so he can hear lower noises; his blood flow moves to his muscles ready to run; his breathing and heart rate increase; he is ready to move. If, however, the snake is at his feet, as per Stephen Porges' Polyvagal theory (2011), Humpty experiences a neuroception not just of danger but of life-threat. He then drops into an emergency parasympathetic brake or freeze experience where he cannot move until it is safe to do so. In both states, to different degrees, Humpty loses concurrent awareness of his senses in a way that decreases accurate perception of his environment.

At a neurological level, Humpty's 'bottom up' automatic unconscious senses switch into action (Rushworth et al. 2002), and, in life-threat freeze, his conscious 'top down' sense-making may go offline (Hopfinger, Buonocore, and Mangun 2000). He may also narrow his view to detailed perception (and memory) of key elements of the situation associated with survival. The duration of this 'offline' time is affected by the degree of overwhelm and whether it is possible to make sense of this situation. If the 'snake' on the path ended up just being a stick, the senses would all come back online, a sense of coherence would be restored and Humpty, on his bushwalk, could begin looking forward to the view again.

Any discussion of sensation needs to remain aware that the accuracy and breadth of sensation are influenced by experiences of threat. These threats can be both physical and subjective, as one stakeholder noted:

> I feel threatened most if I feel that my safety, like my body's safety is in jeopardy. But I feel just as threatened if someone's disrespecting my identity. (ia[1])

The whole person *sense of safety* framework proposed in this book has 'sense of' as a key element of whole person understanding. This intentionally places Humpty's inner sensory experience as a central part of any assessment process. It makes Humpty the final arbiter of what is going on – not external observer classification systems. The complex appraisal process integrating Humpty's perception, attention and subjective experiences are summed up in the simple words 'sense of'. They are a kind of internal ancient trade language that connects and communicates.

When we care for Humpty, we are interested in asking: What is Humpty's 'sense of' his own experience? What is he already appraising? What are his senses communicating to him and to other people around him? How is what he senses linked to the present or the past? Are there any blocks or distortions that impact his capacity to sense his inner or outer worlds accurately? What can the practitioner sense with Humpty? Or reflect back to him to help him 'make sense' of his story and experiences? These questions are important to the generalist seeking to care for the whole person. What follows in this chapter is a philosophical and practical explanation of why those who care for distress could highly value sensing as an integrative and relational whole person experience.

Sensing as integrative communication

The processes of 'sensing' and 'making sense' are interconnected. They link reason and emotion, thought and bodily experiences, environment and inner experience. Sensing includes neural inputs from perception of the environment, as well as inner integrative pattern recognition based on past experience and meanings. The origin of the word 'sense' reveals this link between reason or meaning and body: it comes from the Latin *sensus* meaning 'sensation, feeling, meaning' and *sentiō* ('feel, perceive'), as well as the Old Frankish *sinn* ('reason, judgement, way, direction') and Proto-Germanic *sinnaz* ('mind, meaning') (Wordsense

2020). Its definition includes perceiving via the sense organs, a conscious rationality, an impression, a motivating or discerning awareness, a sound and practical mental capacity, a comprehension, an automatic detection and a wisdom (Wordsense 2020; Merriam Webster 2020). Sensory awareness is an integrative way to understand distress (Barrett et al. 2004).

Senses 'are systems organised to enable us to obtain information about the world' (Marks 2014, 40). Our bodily senses and our sense-making interpretation of those senses are so intertwined it is difficult to define or separate them (Laird and Lacasse 2014, Marks 2014, 3) – there is a constant flow of communication between sensation (or bodily arousal) and cognition (Laird and Lacasse 2014) – including feelings, 'cognitive emotion' or 'hot thought' (Thagard 2008). Sensing concurrently attends to many aspects of Humpty. Both positivist (observed) and post-positivist (experienced) information is integrated and interpreted. Sensing is a key element of any complex system (Kurtz and Snowden 2003). It requires a wide awareness and interconnectedness, as well as an openness to new information, in order to remain accurate. It is a process of connecting, organising and discerning both internal and external environments.

Even when he is unwell, Humpty's experiences are interconnected:

> Illness is an integral experience that can only be artificially reflected into biological, psychological, social and spiritual dimensions.
>
> (Tresolini 1994, 15)

He also senses in an interconnected way across time through memories and his body:

> Experiences remain with us, not only as thought and conscious memories, but also as part of our embodiment. We may mentally and consciously forget, but our body remembers; what we have experienced is both imprinted and expressed in our bodies. Experiences are inextricably subjective phenomena, which are expressed in some way or other, but not necessarily, and most often not, in a straightforward way.
>
> (Kirkengen and Thornquist 2012, 1098)

Sensing is a kind of *gestalt*, a kind of unity (Marks 2014), a perception of the whole, not just a bodily reaction to environment. Early thinkers described all senses as models of touch (Democritus 5th Century BC) or described a 'sensus communis' – that integrated the activity of many senses – 'amidst the diversity of sensory perception there is unity' (Marks 2014, 2). An 'integrated nervous system' (Damasio 1998) links 'factual knowledge and bioregulatory states' (Bechara, Damasio, and Damasio 2000, 296). This involves sophisticated processes of oscillation and synchrony at a neural level (Engel, Fries, and Singer 2001). Rather than simplistic linear 'perception-cognition-action' understanding of sensation, neurobiologists propose an understanding of a 'real-time' (Koziol, Budding, and Chidekel 2011, 772) adaptive continuous integrative 'sensorimotor interaction between a person and his/her environment' (Koziol, Budding, and Chidekel 2011, 786). Other processes that are linked to or rely on this whole person experience of 'sensing' are assessing, appraising, detecting, noticing, recognising, attending, attuning, concordancing and connecting.

This real-time sensory assessment could be a way to understand 'self-rated health', which integrates conscious and unconscious forms of 'sensing' or knowing. The remarkable ability of a person to assess their own health accurately is a relatively underutilised way to understand wellbeing. It is an integrative assessment at the 'cross-road between the social world and psychological experiences on the one hand and the biological world on the other' (Jylhä 2009, 308). A gestalt of sensory integration may underpin this surprisingly accurate way to predict health (Picard, Juster, and Sabiston 2013).

Awareness of the importance of sensation and perception is already part of everyday understanding of fields such as teaching, early childhood, and rehabilitation sciences – where the concepts of 'sensory processing' or 'sensory modulation' are an essential part of research, practice and integrative understanding of the whole (Ben-Sasson et al. 2009, Koziol, Budding, and Chidekel 2011, Kinnealey, Koenig, and Smith 2011). Unfortunately, sensing is still not highly valued in biomedical settings – discredited by assumptions of the body's fallibility and archaic disconnected views of the rational mind as a separate from the body (and therefore more reliable) (Barnacle 2001). This view of the 'silent body and the speaking mind' (Kirkengen and Thornquist 2012, 1097) has led to the subjective experience and voice of the patient being excluded from many diagnostic processes in favour of what has been considered the more objective clinician's appraisal of the situation. And yet the clinician uses his or her senses in every encounter.

Sensing the whole person: From the cellular to the communal

Examining the use of the language and the meaning of 'sense' finds a natural use of this ordinary word across different aspects of being human – from the cellular to the communal. If practitioners could understand the range of sensory inputs and the purpose of sensing, it may contribute to a coherent framework for whole person wellbeing.

Cellular descriptions of 'sensing' include intracellular 'mitochondrial oxygen sensing' (Bell, Emerling, and Chandel 2005), nutrient sensing (Sekine et al. 1994) and the innate immune 'sense of danger' (Hato and Dagher 2015) from non-self (infection) or damaged self (tissue injury). This is described as a 'highly sophisticated sentinel system' (Hato and Dagher 2015, 1459) that includes antibodies, pentraxins (e.g., C-reactive protein), the complement system, immune cells (macrophages, dendritic and killer cells) and epithelial cells (that produce cytokines and chemokines). Immune researchers also note what they have termed 'pattern-recognition receptors' that are have specific recognition processes that are part of innate immunity (Kawai and Akira 2010).

Other *bodily processes* of 'sensing' occur through utilising smell, taste, touch, sight and hearing, as well as proprioception (awareness of the position and movement of the body) and interoception (sense of the internal state of the body).[2] The research into interoception – 'visceral sensing' (Cameron 2001) – is revealing a sophisticated internal homeostatic mechanism that 'senses and integrates signals from inside the body' (Khalsa and Lapidus 2016, 121). These interoceptive sensory feedback processes occur in all systems involved in homeostasis – cardiovascular, pulmonary, gastrointestinal, genitourinary, nociceptive, chemosensory, osmotic, thermoregulatory, visceral, immune and autonomic nervous systems (Khalsa et al. 2018). Interoception has been linked to socio-emotional competence and psychopathology and includes both implicit (subconscious) and explicit (conscious) perception (Murphy et al. 2017). The endocrine, immune and neurological systems are also sophisticated sensory systems with built-in self-regulation and feedback loops. The gastrointestinal system and the organs of the skin and heart are also examples of exquisite sensory systems attuned to micro-fluctuations in nutrients, flora, temperature and oxygenation. They are also attuned to psychosocial cues in order to prepare for future energy and action needs.

Sensation of pain is also an attuned process linked to detecting threat – using nociceptive receptors linked to the rest of the organism in order to activate self-protective systems and behaviours. Pain appraises for physical threat, but in hypervigilance, it can become a threatening experience in its own right. Awareness of safe attachment figures can decrease the vigilance of this system (Crombez et al. 1999, Denison, Åsenlöf, and Lindberg 2004, Eisenberger et al. 2011, Meredith et al. 2006). *Sense of safety* affects pain experiences.

Neurodevelopmental researchers name threat detection, emotion regulation and reward anticipation systems that are part of the human neurological sensory architecture (Teicher et al. 2016), while attention researchers name the Core Response Network that comprises the autonomic nervous system, emotion motor system, limbic system and reticular activating system that 'responds quickly to arousing and threatening stimuli with little input from higher cortical evaluative processes' (Payne, Levine, and Crane-Godreau 2015, para 13).

There is a growing literature around the integrative role of the part of the brain called the insula in appraising internal and external sensory information (including emotion) (Nguyen et al. 2016, Simmons et al. 2013), in interpreting the salience or meaning of that sensation (Wiech et al. 2010) and in mediating awareness (Craig and Craig 2009). The insula has been described as being able to 'integrate perceptions, emotions, thoughts and plans into one subjective image of "our world"' (Kurth et al. 2010, 519). It has been described as offering 'functional organisation and functional connectivity' (Simmons et al. 2013) and has also been mapped to have olfacto-gustatory, cognitive, sensorimotor and social-emotional regions that are distinct and overlap (Kurth et al. 2010). This research adds to the importance of attending to the 'sense of' experiences of both practitioner and person in distress.

Emotions are a form of sensing (e.g., 'sense of sadness' or 'sense of joy') and, when considered in this way, are much more than 'moods'; they are embodied sensory experiences, internal forms of communication. The core emotion of disgust (Panksepp 1982) is even described in terms that link it to the sense of taste. Anxiety, commonly conceptualised as simply a mood disorder, can be conceptualised as an appraisal (or sensation) of threat – an 'amygdala-cortical alarm' (Liddell et al. 2005), a 'reaction to helplessness' (Freud 1979, 327) or 'signal for help' (Freud 1979, 327). Those who study emotion link interpretations of emotion (emotional cognition or emotional thought) directly with the sensation of 'somatic states' that include 'internal milieu, visceral and musculoskeletal' aspects of the soma (Bechara, Damasio, and Damasio 2000, 295). Somatic 'markers' or 'signals', for example, heart rate and skin conductance (Crone et al. 2004), can reveal these internal processes.

Inner spiritual or existential experiences can also be seen as a form of sensing (e.g., sense of peace, sense of despair). Senses can refer to the past (e.g., 'sense of regret') and to the future (e.g., 'sense of hope'). Intrapsychic descriptions of 'sensing' include 'sense of self' – a noticing of the self – or 'sense of capacity', where internal resources to cope are assessed. Communal sensing can include being comforted or distressed by other people or beyond the range of usual perception to the transcendent (in the form 'revelation' or 'insight') or to the environment (e.g., 'sense of connection to country').

Sensing is also a key part of *relating to others*. Psychophysiological research has described the Social Engagement System, which involves cranial nerves and autonomic nervous system. It involves sensing through awareness and orientation to movement, observation of facial expressions, noticing prosody of voices and assessment of social threat (Porges 2003). This system depends on neurological appraisal of threat or safety named 'neuroception'. As discussed in Humpty's bush walk example, it can appraise 'danger' (activating the sympathetic mobilisation system); 'life-threatening' (activating the unmyelinated vagus to brake, immobilise and 'feign death'); and 'safe' (activating the ventral vagal parasympathetic system and sympathetic system in balance) (Porges 2011, Porges 2007). If safety is sensed, it enables prosocial behaviour, affect regulation and physiological homeostasis (Porges 2007). This capacity to sense social belonging and comfort is a key element of *sense of safety*.

Other processes such as 'resonance' may also describe a form of 'sensing' that is linked to mirror neurone and pheromone sensing between people. Sensing connection includes words and meanings, values and approaches to power and moral roles. Interestingly, the term 'consent' includes Latin words *con* ('to know') and *sentire* ('to feel together') (Pellegrino 2006).

Stress researchers, as mentioned in Chapter Four, confirm the buffering impact of relationships to reduce stress from toxic to 'tolerable' (Shonkoff et al. 2012). Social rejection is sensed at the brain level as pain (Eisenberger and Lieberman 2004), while shame causes physiological stress reactions (Dickerson, Gruenewald, and Kemeny 2004, Lucini et al. 2005), which can be misattributed as a form of self-stigma (Corrigan, Watson, and Barr 2006). Some would describe the bodily sensation of shame as an awareness of 'threat to the social self' (Budden 2009) – a fear of disconnection (Brown 2012, Gruenewald et al. 2004). Understanding shame as a physiological sensation that warns of social disconnection (and that can be misunderstood as personal inadequacy) invites sensorimotor and relational approaches to treatment.

Each of these levels of sensing communicates from the cellular to the communal, as part of the whole person interacting within their relationships and environment. When the various levels of the organism work seamlessly together they often go unnoticed (Hamberger 2004). They offer a gestalt or 'real-time' (Koziol, Budding, and Chidekel 2011, 172) understanding of the whole person's experience moment by moment.

Sensing purposefully protects integrity, connection and coherence

Sensing has a purpose. Humpty needs his senses to navigate a complex changing world and to adapt and respond appropriately. Sensing can offer comfort and sense of connection with others or a sense of threat, dread or overwhelm when you perceive you no longer have capacity to cope. Sensing and appraisal of threat or safety is a whole person experience.

Sensation helps Humpty to attend to his need for integrity, connection to others and coherent understanding of his world. Senses can alert Humpty, and any practitioner caring for him, enabling them to intervene early and respond appropriately from a cellular to communal level. Humpty can attend to bodily threat, including pain (invasion), the subtle social alarm of shame (disconnection) or the existential alarm of hopelessness or confusion (incoherence).

From immune processes to social assessment of facial expressions, humans are constantly vigilant – assessing threat and their capacity to respond to it. Appraising or sensing threat involves embodied intuition, perceptions, senses and cognitions. There are many internal and external experiences – including illness experiences (Hou et al. 2014) – that can contribute to an appraisal of a 'personal experience of danger' (Kirkengen and Thornquist 2012, 1096) or 'endangering other' (Kirkengen and Thornquist 2012, 1096). These drive the human organism to protect integrity 'on all existential levels, from the cellular to that of personhood' (Kirkengen and Thornquist 2012, 1096). Christine Courtois and Julian Ford (2009, 17) named both the 'hyperarousal and hypervigilance in relation to external danger … [and the] internal threat of being unable to self-regulate, self-organise, or draw upon relationships to regain self-integrity'. As well as integrity (Kirkengen and Thornquist 2012), coherence and engagement have already been identified as key elements of wellbeing (Dowrick 2004).

When asking stakeholders in my doctoral research what causes threat, three dynamics emerged as threats: invasion (confrontation, disrespect, violence, intimidation, bullying, racism, injustice and all forms of abuse), disconnection (loneliness, exclusion, loss, abandonment, disengagement, being shamed, disregarded and all forms of neglect), and confusion (confusing relationships, being misheard or misunderstood). Each of these experiences is a fundamental threat to integrity, connection and coherence. Table 5.1 summarises relevant literature and stakeholder responses.

Inability to defend against, flee or manage these threats leaves a person with no sense of capacity to face their world. These systems for assessing or sensing

Table 5.1 What Senses Protect

Protecting	Against	Examples
Integrity	Invasion	physical, chemical, microbial invasion, mitosis (cancer), confrontation, disrespect, violence, intimidation, bullying, physical, sexual and emotional abuse, violations, high expectations, disrespect, injustice, racism, sexism, war, being trapped (freedom invaded).
Connection	Disconnection	loneliness, exclusion, loss, abandonment, preoccupied or absent parent (including hospitalised, incarcerated or intoxicated), disengagement, emotional neglect, physical neglect, 'ghosting', non-verbal emotional abuse, being shamed, objectified, disregarded, marginalised, ignored
Coherence	Confusion	confusing relationships, being misheard or misunderstood, double binds, witnessing others violated, patterns that don't make sense, gaslighting, unsure what or how to manage/cope, ambivalence, secrets, deception, betrayal

Note: Collated using information from Felitti et al. 1998, LeFebvre et al. 2019, Teicher et al. 2016, Lynch 2019.

safety or threat are dynamic, appraising internal and external (including relational) resources and threats. They also attend to reactivated memories and anticipated or imagined threats (Kirkengen and Thornquist 2012, Courtois and Ford 2009). As depicted in Figure 5.1, protecting integrity, connection and coherence builds *sense of safety*.

The literature in this field confirms these sensory priorities. People have an outer focus on navigating the world – they direct attention towards connection to others – as well as an inner attunement to intuitions, guiding values and decision-making (Goleman 2013, 4). Adding to Anna Luise Kirkengen and Eline Thornquist's framework (2012), threat can be understood as external (physical, chemical, thermal, microbial or relational), internalised social (social humiliation and scorn) and internal (shame, powerlessness and internal disregard, mitotic, autoimmune, memorial or existential). Maslow named the threat of 'chronic thwarting of basic needs' (Maslow 1954, 77). Confirming the salience of integrity, connection and coherence, he drew attention to 'the general integrity of the organism, basic mastery of the world and ultimate values' (Maslow 1954, 80).

This natural intuitive process of appraisal, or sensing 'what is going on', is an everyday experience that both Humpty and those that care for him experience every day. As will be discussed in later chapters, sensing can be ignored (not attending to communications from the senses), misunderstood (interpreted or perceived incorrectly) or inaccurate (hypersensitive or numbed). It is an ordinary life

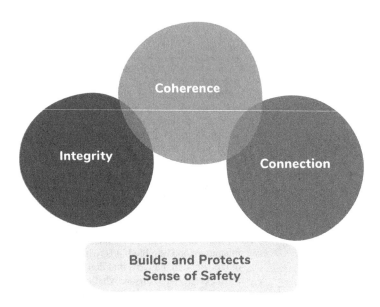

Figure 5.1 What senses protect: From the cellular to the communal.

skill that can be honed and attuned to become more accurate, attentive, perceptive and wise. It involves observation, interpretation, discernment, pattern recognition, meaning-making and wisdom (sense-making) that is open to change moment by moment. Appraisal of threat is also linked to awareness of social or physiological capacity to respond to the threat. It has similarities, too, to good quality whole person assessment, whether in the clinical encounter, school room or boardroom. Accurate sensory appraisal systems are part of building *sense of safety*.

Sensing as a therapeutic skill

Sensing is a key skill of the clinician, the researcher and, of course, the patient, yet it is often still relegated to the art (not the science) of medicine (Malterud 2001). Primary care researcher Trisha Greenhalgh, although still using the slightly dismissive word 'hunch' to describe the clinician's sense of something, seeks to dispel this myth:

> Intuition is not unscientific. It is a highly creative process fundamental to hypothesis generation in science. The experienced practitioner should generate and follow clinical hunches as well as (not instead of) applying the deductive principles of evidence based medicine.
>
> (Greenhalgh 2002, 395)

Interestingly, intuition has been described as: 'affectively charged judgments that arise through rapid, non-conscious, and holistic associations' (Dane and Pratt 2007, 40) – a sensing and discerning of the whole. Skilled reflective practitioners have increasingly accurate intuition, as they are able to attend to and reflect on their own sensory perceptions during decision-making. Ironically, a practitioner's attuned senses may make their scientific observations and acumen more accurate. Reflective practice includes a capacity to manage attention and can be taught and honed (Stange, Peigorsh, and Miller 2003). Torbert describes four types of attention, which could also describe 'knowing' in the primary care setting: 'intuitive knowing of purposes, intellectual knowing of strategy, embodied sensuous knowing of one's behaviour, and an empirical knowing of the outside world' (Reason and Bradbury 2001, 12). Maintaining the capacity to attend to or sense multiple forms of knowledge is a key skill of the generalist (Epstein 2017).

Sensing and sense-making are key skills of a wise clinician (Reeve 2019). Practitioners who are able to attune to and interpret their own senses and perceptions offer a sophisticated capacity to hold a wide view and interpret accurately. They can learn to attend to senses while discerning their accuracy and relevance for clinical appraisal and decision-making.

Sense of safety: A reasonable response to threat

If, as we have explored, *sense of safety* is an overarching need, and sensing has a purpose to protect integrity, connection and coherence, then *loss of sense of safety* caused by many different forms of threat (not just 'trauma') will impact wellbeing of the whole person. This means that any defences against *loss of sense of safety* are deeply logical, and important. Whole person care involves being able to acknowledge the many ways that our physiological and relational systems can become dysregulated by and defensive towards threat.

Not all threat is pathogenic, as Selye (1956) noted in his term 'eustress'. Instead, only threat that is appraised as overwhelming the individual's capacity to adapt causes long term impacts and activation of defences. Threat causes 'complex interactions of physiological, emotional and cognitive experiences that result in loss of *sense of safety*. This process is a relational one with interactions at every level' (Whiting et al. 2012, 30)(italics added). Defence and safety systems are 'information organising systems' that impact biological patterns, social behaviour and the maturation of self-constructs (Gilbert 1993, 131).

Threat to *sense of safety* activates fight, flight or freeze mechanisms and may underlie pathological processes such as rigidity, chaos, avoidance, fragmentation, incoherence, instability, low self-esteem, addiction,[3] escape, distraction, vigilance, self-harm and suicidality. Though the term is not used directly, *loss* (or reduction or absence) *of sense of safety* is also implied in discussions of defences, stress, fear, threat, trauma, helplessness, alarm, flooding, nociception, nocebo, negative valence, avoidance, hypervigilance and even coping and resilience. These are ordinary terms that reveal the pattern. They are descriptions of the everyday human experience of *loss of sense of safety*.

Terms that mean the opposite of *sense of safety* are also relevant, such as 'sense of threat', 'health-related threat' (Hou et al. 2014) or 'sense of danger' (including the immunological understanding of 'sense of danger' (Matzinger 2002)) already mentioned. Phenomenologist Heidegger described a pattern of unease, or *unheimlich*, translated as 'not at home' (Capobianco 2005), while others describe a sense of alienation – 'being ill is above all alienation from the world' (Buytendijk 1974). All these terms enrich our understanding of the concept of *loss of sense of safety*.

Understanding defences is of practical importance as practitioners seek to understand health behaviours and treatment 'resistance', as well as seemingly incoherent choices such as addictions, risk-taking or conflict in the playground or workplace. Freud suggested that anticipation of danger is a rational 'linchpin' (Sampson 1990, 115) underlying defences and that behaviour can be 'transfigured in a rational light' (1926, 146) if understood as a defensive reaction.

In a Canadian psychiatric setting, Robert Maunder and Jon Hunter (2016, 10) note: 'Feeling secure in a frightening circumstance is often perceived as a more urgent goal than remaining healthy over a longer time'. Defences function to control anxiety (Cramer 2000) and therefore 'the patient's customary way of dealing with stress may interfere with their following treatment advice' (Cramer 2000, 641). William Blatz (1973, 114) called these defences 'deputy agents' that enable a person to avoid feelings of insecurity or inadequacy. As mentioned in the Introduction, distress reduction behaviours or defences are used to manage overwhelming feelings. They are meaningful and purposeful responses to threat that are activated both by realistic danger or perception of danger (Sampson 1990). They are used to cope with 'lack of basic forms of safety' (Courtois and Ford 2009, 91). Awareness of defensive coping systems can help the generalist to attend to the underlying threat and its associated physiological and psychological dysregulation. Rather than focus on treatment of the defence or labelling a comorbid 'disorder', practitioners can attend to the underlying *loss of sense of safety*.

As many defences are subjective experiences, their integration into understandings of distress in primary health has been delayed (Northoff et al. 2007). Addictive, obsessive, compulsive and avoidant processes seen regularly in primary care are forms of defence. Rather than comorbidity – they may be revealing a deeper morbidity – the loss of a subjective experience of safety.

In his important Interpersonal Theory of Psychiatry, Stack Sullivan suggested directing treatment towards the underlying threat in order to facilitate the 'development of a person's living' (Sullivan 1953, 12). He suggests treating threat 'rather than deal[ing] with symptoms called out by anxiety or to avoid anxiety' (Sullivan 1953, 146) – loss of safety or defences against loss of safety. Paul Gilbert, who researches self-compassion as a way to soothe internal threat, recommends becoming aware of what threatens people and how they are responding to it – especially if that response is repetitive (such as avoidance or attack). He promotes 'therapeutic interventions that change avoidance into exploration' (Gilbert 1993, 131). Alan Rappoport identifies:

People unconsciously assess their social environments for signals of safety and danger, relaxing their defences when it seems safe to do so ... in order for the pathological adaptations to be dispensed with, the person must discover that the dangerous situations no longer exist, and that it is now safe to act in healthier ways.

(Rappoport 1997, 250)

This aligns with primary care priorities of seeking to restore 'capacity for living' (Reeve 2018) and reminds us that safety can lead to comfort and courage.

Sense of safety is a meta-need (Maslow 1954); it is an underlying part of health. Threat to *sense of safety* is, then, of fundamental importance to those who seek to see the whole of Humpty. Understanding threat and focusing on building *sense of safety* can help to make it 'safe to act in healthier ways' (Rappoport 1997, 250). *Sense of safety* and *loss of sense of safety*, for both Humpty and his practitioner, can reveal underlying patterns, including dysregulation and defences, that impact the whole person.

Notes

1 ia=indigenous academic stakeholder interviewed as part of PhD (Lynch 2019)
2 This definition of interoception has been refined to include some sensations not strictly internal (such as sensual touch and tickling) that are processed by the same neural pathways as interoceptive signals – these include vagus and glossopharyngeal cranial nerves, and small diameter fibres in the spinothalamic tract (Murphy et al. 2017).
3 Some describe addiction as a response to overwhelm (Volkow et al. 2010).

References

Barnacle, Robyn, ed. 2001. *Phenomenology*. Edited by John Bowden, *Qualitative research methods series*. Melbourne: RMIT University Press.

Barrett, Lisa Feldman, Karen S. Quigley, Eliza Bliss-Moreau, and Keith R. Aronson. 2004. 'Interoceptive sensitivity and self-reports of emotional experience.' *Journal of Personality and Social Psychology* 87 (5):684–697. doi:10.1037/0022-3514.87.5.684.

Bechara, Antoine, Hanna Damasio, and Antonio R. Damasio. 2000. 'Emotion, decision making and the orbitofrontal cortex.' *Cerebral Cortex* 10 (3):295–307.

Bell, Eric L., Brooke M. Emerling, and Navdeep S. Chandel. 2005. 'Mitochondrial regulation of oxygen sensing.' *Mitochondrion* 5 (5):322–332.

Ben-Sasson, Ayelet, Liat Hen, Ronen Fluss, Sharon A Cermak, Batya Engel-Yeger, and Eynat Gal. 2009. 'A meta-analysis of sensory modulation symptoms in individuals with autism spectrum disorders.' *Journal of Autism and Developmental Disorders* 39 (1):1–11.

Blatz, W.E. 1973. 'The theory of human security.' In *Child development: Selected readings*, edited by L.M. Brockman, J.H. Whiteley, and J.P. Zubek, 150–166. Toronto: McClelland and Stewart Ltd.

Brown, Brené. 2012. *Daring greatly: How the courage to be vulnerable transforms the way we live, love, parent, and lead.* United Kingdom: Penguin Random House UK.

Budden, Ashwin. 2009. 'The role of shame in posttraumatic stress disorder: A proposal for a socio-emotional model for DSM-V.' *Social Science & Medicine* 69 (7):1032–1039.

Buytendijk, Frederik J. 1974. *Prolegomena to an anthropological physiology.* Duquesne: University Press, Pittsburgh.

Cameron, Oliver G. 2001. *Visceral sensory neuroscience: Interoception.* Oxford: Oxford University Press.

Capobianco, Richard. 2005. 'Heidegger's turn toward home: On Dasein's primordial relation to being.' *Epoché: A Journal for the History of Philosophy* 10 (1):155–173.

Corrigan, Patrick W., Amy C. Watson, and Leah Barr. 2006. 'The self-stigma of mental illness: Implications for self-esteem and self-efficacy.' *Journal of Social and Clinical Psychology* 25 (8):875–884.

Courtois, C., and Julian Ford, eds. 2009. *Treating complex Traumatic stress. An evidence based guide.* New York: The Guilford Press.

Craig, Arthur D., and A.D. Craig. 2009. 'How do you feel--now? The anterior insula and human awareness.' *Nature Reviews Neuroscience* 10 (1):59–70.

Cramer, Phebe. 2000. 'Defense mechanisms in psychology today: Further processes for adaptation.' *American Psychologist* 55 (6):637–646.

Crombez, Geert, Chris Eccleston, Frank Baeyens, Boudewijn Van Houdenhove, and Annelies Van Den Broeck. 1999. 'Attention to chronic pain is dependent upon pain-related fear.' *Journal of Psychosomatic Research* 47 (5):403–410.

Crone, Eveline A., Riek J.M. Somsen, Bert Van Beek, and Maurits W. Van Der Molen. 2004. 'Heart rate and skin conductance analysis of antecedents and consequences of decision making.' *Psychophysiology* 41 (4):531–540.

Damasio, Antonio R. 1998. 'Emotion in the perspective of an integrated nervous system.' *Brain Research Reviews* 26:83–86.

Dane, Erik, and Michael G. Pratt. 2007. 'Exploring intuition and its role in managerial decision making.' *Academy of Management Review* 32 (1):33–54.

Denison, Eva, P. Åsenlöf, and P. Lindberg. 2004. 'Self-efficacy, fear avoidance, and pain intensity as predictors of disability in subacute and chronic musculoskeletal pain patients in primary health care.' *Pain* 111 (3):245–252.

Dickerson, Sally S., Tara L. Gruenewald, and Margaret E. Kemeny. 2004. 'When the social self is threatened: Shame, physiology, and health.' *Journal of Personality* 72 (6):1191–1216.

Dowrick, C. 2004. *Beyond depression: A new approach to understanding and management.* London: Oxford University Press.

Eisenberger, Naomi I., and Matthew D. Lieberman. 2004. 'Why rejection hurts: A common neural alarm system for physical and social pain.' *Trends in Cognitive Sciences* 8 (7):294–300.

Eisenberger, Naomi I., S.L. Master, and T.K. Inagaki. 2011. 'Attachment figures activate a safety signal-related neural region and reduce pain experience.' *Proceedings of the National Academy of Sciences* 108 (28):11721–11726.

Engel, Andreas K., Pascal Fries, and Wolf Singer. 2001. 'Dynamic predictions: Oscillations and synchrony in top–down processing.' *Nature Reviews Neuroscience* 2 (10):704–716.

Epstein, Ronald. 2017. *Attending: Medicine, mindfulness, and humanity.* New York: Scribner, Simon and Schuster.

Felitti, V.J., R.F. Anda, D. Nordenberg, D.F. Williamson, A.M. Spitz, V. Edwards, M.P. Koss, and J.S. Marks. 1998. 'Relationship of childhood abuse and household dysfunction to many of the leading causes of death in adults: The Adverse Childhood Experiences (ACE) study.' *American Journal of Preventive Medicine* 14 (4):245–258.

Freud, S. 1979. *Sigmund Freud on psychopathology*. Reading: Cox and Wyman Ltd.

Gilbert, Paul. 1993. 'Defence and safety: Their function in social behaviour and psychopathology.' *British Journal of Clinical Psychology* 32 (2):131–153.

Goleman, Daniel. 2013. *Focus: The hidden driver of excellence*. New York: HarperCollins Publishers.

Greenhalgh, T. 2002. 'Intuition and evidence – uneasy bedfellows?' *British Journal of General Practice* 52:395–400.

Gruenewald, Tara L., Margaret E. Kemeny, Najib Aziz, and John L. Fahey. 2004. 'Acute threat to the social self: Shame, social self-esteem, and cortisol activity.' *Psychosomatic Medicine* 66 (6):915–924.

Hamberger, E. 2004. 'Transdisciplinarity: A scientific essential.' *Annals of the New York Academy of Sciences* 1028:487–496. doi:10.1196/annals.1322.039.

Hato, Takashi, and Pierre C. Dagher. 2015. 'How the innate immune system senses trouble and causes trouble.' *Clinical Journal of the American Society of Nephrology* 10 (8):1459–1469.

Hopfinger, Joseph B., Michael H. Buonocore, and George R. Mangun. 2000. 'The neural mechanisms of top-down attentional control.' *Nature Neuroscience* 3 (3):284–291.

Hou, Ruihua, Rona Moss-Morris, Anna Risdale, Jeannette Lynch, Preshan Jeevaratnam, Brendan P. Bradley, and Karin Mogg. 2014. 'Attention processes in chronic fatigue syndrome: Attentional bias for health-related threat and the role of attentional control.' *Behaviour Research and Therapy* 52:9–16.

Jylhä, Marja. 2009. 'What is self-rated health and why does it predict mortality? Towards a unified conceptual model.' *Social Science & Medicine* 69 (3):307–316.

Kawai, Taro, and Shizuo Akira. 2010. 'The role of pattern-recognition receptors in innate immunity: Update on Toll-like receptors.' *Nature Immunology* 11 (5):373–384.

Khalsa, Sahib S., Ralph Adolphs, Oliver G. Cameron, Hugo D. Critchley, Paul W. Davenport, Justin S. Feinstein, Jamie D. Feusner, Sarah N. Garfinkel, Richard D. Lane, and Wolf E. Mehling. 2018. 'Interoception and mental health: A roadmap.' *Biological Psychiatry: Cognitive Neuroscience and Neuroimaging* 3 (6):501–513.

Khalsa, Sahib S., and Rachel C. Lapidus. 2016. 'Can interoception improve the pragmatic search for biomarkers in psychiatry?' *Frontiers in Psychiatry* 7:1–19. https://doi.org/10.3389/fpsyt.2016.00121.

Kinnealey, Moya, Kristie Patten Koenig, and Sinclair Smith. 2011. 'Relationships between sensory modulation and social supports and health-related quality of life.' *American Journal of Occupational Therapy* 65 (3):320–327.

Kirkengen, Anna Luise, and Eline Thornquist. 2012. 'The lived body as a medical topic: An argument for an ethically informed epistemology.' *Journal of Evaluation in Clinical Practice* 18 (5):1095–1101.

Koziol, Leonard F., Deborah Ely Budding, and Dana Chidekel. 2011. 'Sensory integration, sensory processing, and sensory modulation disorders: Putative functional neuroanatomic underpinnings.' *The Cerebellum* 10 (4):770–792.

Kurth, Florian, Karl Zilles, Peter T. Fox, Angela R. Laird, and Simon B. Eickhoff. 2010. 'A link between the systems: Functional differentiation and integration within the human insula revealed by meta-analysis.' *Brain Structure and Function* 214 (5–6):519–534.

Kurtz, Cynthia F., and David J. Snowden. 2003. 'The new dynamics of strategy: Sensemaking in a complex and complicated world.' *IBM Systems Journal* 42 (3):462–483.

Laird, James D., and Katherine Lacasse. 2014. 'Bodily influences on emotional feelings: Accumulating evidence and extensions of William James's theory of emotion.' *Emotion Review* 6 (1):27–34.

LeFebvre, Leah E., Mike Allen, Ryan D. Rasner, Shelby Garstad, Aleksander Wilms, and Callie Parrish. 2019. 'Ghosting in emerging adults' romantic relationships: The digital dissolution disappearance strategy.' *Imagination, Cognition and Personality* 39 (2):125–150.

Liddell, Belinda J., Kerri J. Brown, Andrew H. Kemp, Matthew J. Barton, Pritha Das, Anthony Peduto, Evian Gordon, and Leanne M. Williams. 2005. 'A direct brainstem–amygdala–cortical "alarm" system for subliminal signals of fear.' *Neuroimage* 24 (1):235–243.

Lucini, Daniela, Gaetana Di Fede, Gianfranco Parati, and Massimo Pagani. 2005. 'Impact of chronic psychosocial stress on autonomic cardiovascular regulation in otherwise healthy subjects.' *Hypertension* 46 (5):1201–1206.

Lynch, J.M. 2019. *Sense of safety: A whole person approach to distress.* PhD, Primary Care Clinical Unit, University of Queensland.

Malterud, Kirsti. 2001. 'The art and science of clinical knowledge: Evidence beyond measures and numbers.' *The Lancet* 358 (9279):397–400.

Marks, Lawrence E. 2014. *The unity of the senses: Interrelations among the modalities, cognition and perception.* New York: Academic Press.

Maslow, A.H. 1954. *Motivation and personality third edition.* Edited by R. Frager, J. Fadiman, C. McReynolds, and R. Cox. New York: Harper Collins Publishers.

Matzinger, Polly. 2002. 'The danger model: A renewed sense of self.' *Science* 296 (5566):301–305.

Maunder, Robert G., and Jonathan J. Hunter. 2016. 'Can patients be "attached" to healthcare providers? An observational study to measure attachment phenomena in patient–provider relationships.' *BMJ Open* 6 (5):e011068. doi:10.1136/bmjopen-2016-011068.

Meredith, Pamela, Jenny Strong, and Judith A. Feeney. 2006. 'Adult attachment, anxiety, and pain self-efficacy as predictors of pain intensity and disability.' *Pain* 123 (1):146–154.

Merriam Webster online. 2020. Springfield, MA: Merriam-Webster.

Murphy, Jennifer, Rebecca Brewer, Caroline Catmur, and Geoffrey Bird. 2017. 'Interoception and psychopathology: A developmental neuroscience perspective.' *Developmental Cognitive Neuroscience* 23:45–56.

Nguyen, Vinh Thai, Michael Breakspear, Xintao Hu, and Christine Cong Guo. 2016. 'The integration of the internal and external milieu in the insula during dynamic emotional experiences.' *Neuroimage* 124:455–463.

Northoff, Georg, Felix Bermpohl, Frank Schoeneich, and Heinz Boeker. 2007. 'How does our brain constitute defense mechanisms? First-person neuroscience and psychoanalysis.' *Psychotherapy and Psychosomatics* 76 (3):141–153.

Panksepp, Jaak. 1982. 'Toward a general psychobiological theory of emotions.' *Behavioral and Brain Sciences* 5 (3):407–422.

Payne, Peter, Peter A. Levine, and Mardi A. Crane-Godreau. 2015. 'Somatic experiencing: Using interoception and proprioception as core elements of trauma therapy.' *Frontiers in Psychology* 6 (93). https://doi.org/10.3389/fpsyg.2015.00093.

Pellegrino, Edmund D. 2006. 'Toward a reconstruction of medical morality.' *The American Journal of Bioethics* 6 (2):65–71.

Picard, Martin, Robert-Paul Juster, and Catherine M. Sabiston. 2013. 'Is the whole greater than the sum of the parts? Self-rated health and transdisciplinarity.' *Health* 5:24–30. doi:10.4236/health.2013.512A004.

Porges, Stephen W. 2003. 'Social engagement and attachment.' *Annals of the New York Academy of Sciences* 1008 (1):31–47.

Porges, Stephen W. 2007. 'The polyvagal perspective.' *Biological Psychology* 74 (2):116–143.

Porges, Stephen W. 2011. *The polyvagal theory: Neurophysiological foundations of emotions, attachment, communication, and self-regulation.* New York: W.W. Norton & Company.

Rappoport, Alan. 1997. 'The patient's search for safety: The organizing principle in psychotherapy.' *Psychotherapy: Theory, Research, Practice, Training* 34 (3):250–261.

Reason, Peter, and Hilary Bradbury. 2001. *Handbook of action research: Participative Inquiry and Practice.* London: Sage.

Reeve, Joanne. 2018. 'Scholarship-based medicine: Teaching tomorrow's generalists why it's time to retire EBM.' *British Journal of General Practice* 68 (673):390–391.

Reeve, Joanne. 2019. 'Wise GP: Championing the Bananarama principle in general practice.' Accessed 25/2/20. https://www.rcgp.org.uk/clinical-and-research/about/clinical-news/2019/october/wise-gp-championing-the-bananarama-principle-in-general-practice.aspx.

Rushworth, M.F.S., K.A. Hadland, T. Paus, and P.K. Sipila. 2002. 'Role of the human medial frontal cortex in task switching: A combined fMRI and TMS study.' *Journal of Neurophysiology* 87 (5):2577–2592.

Sampson, Harold. 1990. 'How the patient's sense of danger and safety influence the analytic process.' *Psychoanalytic Psychology* 7 (1):115–124.

Sekine, Nobuo, Vincenzo Cirulli, Romano Regazzi, Laura J. Brown, Elena Gine, Jorge Tamarit-Rodriguez, Milena Girotti, Sandrine Marie, Michael J. MacDonald, and Claes B. Wollheim. 1994. 'Low lactate dehydrogenase and high mitochondrial glycerol phosphate dehydrogenase in pancreatic beta-cells. Potential role in nutrient sensing.' *Journal of Biological Chemistry* 269 (7):4895–4902.

Selye, Hans. 1956. *The stress of life.* New York: McGraw Hill Book Company.

Shonkoff, Jack P., Andrew S. Garner, Benjamin S. Siegel, Mary I. Dobbins, Marian F. Earls, Laura McGuinn, John Pascoe, David L. Wood, and Committee on Psychosocial Aspects of Child, Family Health, Adoption Committee on Early Childhood, and Dependent Care. 2012. 'The lifelong effects of early childhood adversity and toxic stress.' *Pediatrics* 129 (1):e232–e246.

Simmons, W. Kyle, Jason A. Avery, Joel C. Barcalow, Jerzy Bodurka, Wayne C. Drevets, and Patrick Bellgowan. 2013. 'Keeping the body in mind: Insula functional organization and functional connectivity integrate interoceptive, exteroceptive, and emotional awareness.' *Human Brain Mapping* 34 (11):2944–2958.

Stange, Kurt C., Karen M. Peigorsh, and William L. Miller. 2003. 'Commentary: Reflective practice.' *Families, Systems, & Health* 21 (1):24–27.

Sullivan, Harry Stack. 1953. *The interpersonal theory of psychiatry.* Edited by H. Swick Perry, and M. Ladd Gawel. London: Tavistock Publications Ltd.

Teicher, Martin H., Jacqueline A. Samson, Carl M. Anderson, and Kyoko Ohashi. 2016. 'The effects of childhood maltreatment on brain structure, function and connectivity.' *Nature Reviews Neuroscience* 17 (10):652–666.

Thagard, Paul. 2008. *Hot thought: Mechanisms and applications of emotional cognition.* London: The MIT Press.

Tresolini, CP. 1994. 'Health professions education and relationship-centered care.' In *Pew-Fetzer task report*. San Francisco: Pew Health Professions Commission.

Volkow, Nora D., Gene-Jack Wang, Joanna S. Fowler, Dardo Tomasi, Frank Telang, and Ruben Baler. 2010. 'Addiction: Decreased reward sensitivity and increased expectation sensitivity conspire to overwhelm the brain's control circuit.' *Bioessays* 32 (9):748–755.

Whiting, Jason B., Douglas B. Smith, Megan Oka, and Gunnur Karakurt. 2012. 'Safety in intimate partnerships: The role of appraisals and threat.' *Journal of Family Violence* 27 (4):313–320.

Wiech, Katja, Chia-shu Lin, Kay H. Brodersen, Ulrike Bingel, Markus Ploner, and Irene Tracey. 2010. 'Anterior insula integrates information about salience into perceptual decisions about pain.' *Journal of Neuroscience* 30 (48):16324–16331.

Wordsense. 2020. 'Online dictionary Wordsense.eu.' Accessed 27/1/20. https://www.wordsense.eu/sensus/.

Section Two

Building the concept of *sense of safety*

Insights from consultation

Building on the first section, Section Two takes the reader on a journey through the findings from stakeholder consultations, academic critique and analysis of transdisciplinary literature that were part of my doctoral research (Lynch 2019). This doctoral research, undertaken in Australia, used a transdisciplinary generalist methodology (Lynch et al. 2020).

Stakeholder consultation was conducted in three stages: initial question (to be discussed in this Chapter Six), follow up questions (included in following chapters) and reflection on iterations of the research findings (included in Chapter Ten). As outlined in the Introduction, stakeholders included people with lived experience of being patients (le), rural and urban general practitioners (gp), indigenous Australian Aboriginal academics (ia) and multidisciplinary mental health clinicians (mhc). The ideas were also submitted for formal academic review to a ten-member international multidisciplinary academic panel (denoted as mhc-a, and gp-a), which will be discussed in Chapter Ten.

In this section you will be introduced to the analysis of this research. Analysis of the data included iterative and reflexive (Tobin and Begley 2004) coding and the development of theoretical or pattern codes through inductive, deductive and abductive reasoning, the use of Inclusive Logic and discernment (Crabtree and Miller 1999, Nicolescu 2014).

The concept of *sense of safety* will be discussed in Section Two as an active appraisal process that includes a broad scope of attention (*whole person domains*) and concurrent processes (*sense of safety dynamics*) that build, protect and reveal wellbeing. Learning to attend to the broad scope and dynamics of *sense of safety* is something that both the practitioner and Humpty can do to restore their own and other's wellbeing.

References

Crabtree, Benjamin F., and William L. Miller. 1999. *Doing qualitative research*. Thousand Oaks, CA: Sage publications.

Lynch, J.M. 2019. *Sense of safety: A whole person approach to distress*. PhD, Primary Care Clinical Unit, University of Queensland.

Lynch, J.M., C.F. Dowrick, Pamela Meredith, S.L.T. McGregor, and Mieke Van Driel. 2020. 'Transdisciplinary generalism: Naming the epistemology and philosophy of the generalist.' *Journal of Evaluation in Clinical Practice*, 1–10.

Nicolescu, Basarab. 2014. 'Methodology of transdisciplinarity.' *World Futures* 70 (3–4):186–199.

Tobin, Gerard A., and Cecily M. Begley. 2004. 'Methodological rigour within a qualitative framework.' *Journal of Advanced Nursing* 48 (4):388–396.

6 The integrative gift of an ordinary phrase – Humpty's native tongue

- The ordinary English phrase 'sense of safety' offers a genuine shared language for communication about wellbeing
- The phrase 'sense of safety' implies a broad concurrent awareness of self, other and context
- Appraising a 'sense of safety' is an active process of knowing

'Sense of safety' is an ordinary English phrase, but does it communicate clearly and have a communal shared understanding? Is it an adequate trade language that unites the different knowledge cultures? Does the phrase 'sense of safety' enable understanding of the complex whole person? When people use the English phrase 'sense of safety', what do they mean?

As an initial stage of focus groups and interviews, before we had done more than introduce ourselves, I asked stakeholders to write down their answer to this key question:

What does the phrase 'sense of safety' mean to you?

Fundamentally, this question sought to see whether the ordinary English phrase 'sense of safety' was a widely understood phrase and whether the meaning across descriptions was coherent and shared enough to be useful: was 'sense of safety' a natural, understandable part of Humpty's native tongue? What emerged from the written responses did more than establish the joint understanding of the term. It also revealed a *concurrent breadth of perception* and an *active appraisal process* that underpinned sensing safety.

Breadth of perception: *what* contributes to *sense of safety*?

When stakeholders described the meaning of 'sense of safety', their descriptions included multiple layers of awareness – across *self, other* and *context*.

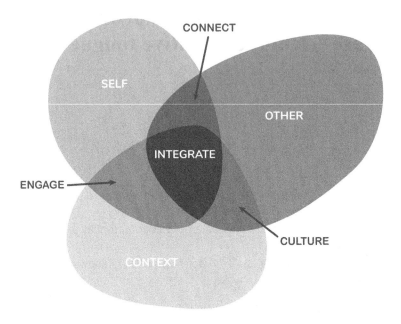

Figure 6.1 Broad concurrent awareness: mapping responses to 'What does the phrase "sense of safety" mean to you?'

Often all three were mentioned at once. They also described dynamic awareness of experiences of self-in-relation to other (named 'connect'); self-in-relation to context (named 'engage') and others-in-relation to their context (named 'culture'). These key elements are mapped in Figure 6.1. This *broad awareness* of the 'whole' of what was going on at that moment was a consistent finding across descriptions. It revealed not only the breadth of information appraised to determine a 'sense of safety', but also the concurrent awareness of many aspects of safety at once.

Perception of *self* included an appraisal of capacity to face (or 'engage') threat, experience in relationships (safety to 'connect') and sense of freedom to be and own themselves. They described sensory and cognitive experiences of threat, and used words such as 'anxiety', 'fear', 'vulnerability', 'intimidation', being 'threatened', 'harmed' or 'compromised'.

Perception of *others* included awareness of other people's availability, and presence – assessing 'connection'. They also assessed character (e.g., 'trustworthy'), and subjective observations, interpretations and perceptions of behaviour. They frequently mentioned awareness of themselves in relationship to or in the presence of another person. This relational assessment included many descriptions of feelings of belonging, trust, respect and acceptance with others. They also described their sense of freedom to express themselves and be themselves in the presence of the other, as well as feeling safe in culture.

Perception of *context* included awareness of place or situation over time (including future 'demands', 'expectations', 'consequences' or 'impact'). They mentioned safety being affected by work and living environments, culture, time, information, opportunity and needs being met. When noticing themselves in relation to context, they noted their own confidence to 'engage' with their context, aware of their own capacity to face threat, including a sense of relational support.

As well as awareness of self, other and context, there were descriptions of an integrative appraisal process – allowing concurrent real-time active attention to the whole. Somehow information from self, other and context is 'known' all at once, giving a 'sense of safety' in that moment – depicted as 'integrate' where these aspects intersect in Figure 6.1. Stakeholder descriptions repeatedly revealed concurrent awareness: broad integrative attention to time, connections, context, relationships, identity, agency, culture and moment-by-moment emotional and bodily experiences.

Active appraisal process: *how* is safety sensed?

Active appraisal process: **sense of safety** *– broad concurrent awareness*

Appraisal of 'sense of safety' is an active process. Stakeholder descriptions repeatedly used verbs to describe a process of appraisal that included feeling, sensing, owning and being when they described 'sense of safety'. Appraisal of *sense of safety* emerged as an active process, stakeholders were aware of dynamics between self, other and context and of the degree of threat and their own sense of capacity.

Those who write about the appraisal process involved in clinical assessment describe 'diagnosis' as a verb or procedure, not a denotation (Sadler 2005). Similarly, those who study professional knowledge see 'knowing' as a verb, not a noun (Carlsen, Von Krogh, and Klev 2004) – an active reflective process, rather than a static piece of evidence. Seeing clinical appraisal (or diagnosis) as an active process counters the narrow interpretation of diagnosis as classification (Langeland et al. 2007). As an active relational process that includes awareness of the self, other and context, diagnosis becomes more personal. It becomes less a societal contract (Blazer 2005) that endorses 'abdication of responsibility' (Carey and Pilgrim 2010, 449) or the individualisation of health responsibility (Yoder 2002). Instead, it aligns with Sadler's journey-like description of diagnosis as a 'consistent way to forge clinical understanding and moral purpose into therapeutic action' (Sadler 2005, 419). Appraisal of one's own safety aligns with clinical appraisal – they are a moment-by-moment active dynamic kind of 'knowing'. Sensing safety is a kind of self-diagnosis.

Active appraisal process: **sense of safety** *– sensory embodied experience*

Stakeholder responses revealed an active moment-by-moment bodily and sensory appraisal of 'sense of safety'. Occasionally responses used cognitive processes (e.g., 'without negative consequences' (mhc)), but, overwhelmingly, descriptions used emotional and sensory verbs to describe the process of appraisal. One participant described it as a 'state of feeling' (mhc). Although the word 'sense' was only used four times in the 37 written descriptions, words such as 'be' or 'being' were used 16 times, and 'feel' or 'feeling' were used 34 times. These active sensory words used by each stakeholder group (GPs, indigenous academics, patients and mental health clinicians) reveal an ongoing embodied process of appraisal, not merely a cognitive observation of a static state or experience. They document an active role of the participant in the process of noticing and assessing safety and 'being' safe, not merely a passive observer or consumer. One person described 'sense of safety' as 'a feeling of wellbeing and calm and belonging without fear/anxiety' (mhc). Other embodied experiences were expressed in as a very personal and even spiritual awareness of the safety of the self. They also described their sense of agency, directed movement and their sense of having a voice.

Active appraisal process: sense of safety – *dynamic and relational*

Descriptions of the phrase 'sense of safety' repeatedly mentioned awareness of time. They mentioned awareness of threat from the past, moment-by-moment awareness of the present and consideration of the risk of ongoing harm or hope into the future. Awareness of time, place, environment and culture, as well as dynamic awareness of relationships (even those not currently present), was part of most descriptions of the meaning of 'sense of safety'. This active awareness, open to changing information, aware of time passing and people coming and going, aware of risk shifting, growing or diminishing, is a reminder that people are dynamic. Their complexity needs to be described with verbs, not nouns.

Active appraisal process: sense of safety – *integrative gestalt*

Stakeholders simple written descriptions of the meaning to them of the phrase 'sense of safety' gave more than expected. Not only did they seem to have a shared coherent understanding of the term, they described a broad concurrent awareness and dynamic responsive awareness of self, other and context. They described an active perceptive process that included being aware of (noticing) the whole experience and making an overall decision about whether they experienced a *sense of safety*. This process involves sensory perception – active embodied awareness – as well as integrative sense-making.

This awareness also seems to be an integrative kind of *gestalt* – somehow discerning the current overall situation. Perceiving or sensing safety is an integrative process, a reliable individualised way to assess your personal capacity to cope in this particular situation. Of course, as we discussed in Chapter Five, appraisal systems can get dysregulated and may need to be trained to be more accurate. In highly stressful situations such as domestic violence, however, they have proven to be more accurate than other supposedly more accurate measures. According to the research into batterer intervention, 'the most consistent and strongest marker – as useful as the batterer characteristics combined', was the women's 'perceptions of safety' (Gondolf 2002). So, even under pressure, appraisal of *sense of safety* can be reliable and accurate and more coherent or integrative than other ways to measure. It seems this ordinary English phrase has a gift within in it – an embodied, integrative way to see the whole. Humpty does seem to be able to discern his whole in a dynamic reliable way.

Later questioning of stakeholders confirmed these findings, as will be discussed in the following chapters that consider the breadth of awareness – the domains of the whole person that contribute to *sense of safety* (Chapter Seven) – and the dynamic processes involved in building *sense of safety* (Chapter Nine). When an academic clinician was asked to critique the concept of 'sense of safety' as part of my doctoral Advisory Panel, he confirmed that 'sense of safety' is a shared language:

> I think sense of safety is a lovely phrase – it is common English – it works – everyone thinks they know what it means – and probably what everyone's idea of what it means is not too different from what everyone else's idea of what it means – so it is useful. (mhc-a)

This ordinary phrase, built over generations of use between people, seems to be a really important part of Humpty's native tongue, grounded in the senses and in the direction of travel – towards the comfort and courage of safety. Sensing safety concurrently appraises a breadth of self, other and context. It is an active, dynamic, sensory and relational process that offers an integrative *gestalt*. It could help practitioners and Humpty himself to notice the whole person. *Sense of safety* seems to be a phrase that could enliven and encourage paradigm change – towards seeing the dynamic whole person in their real world.

References

Blazer, Dan German. 2005. *The age of melancholy: 'Major depression' and its social origins*. New York: Routledge.

Carey, Timothy A., and David Pilgrim. 2010. 'Diagnosis and formulation: What should we tell the students?' *Clinical Psychology & Psychotherapy* 17 (6):447–454.

Carlsen, Arne, George Von Krogh, and Roger Klev. 2004. *Living knowledge: The dynamics of professional service work*. New York: Palgrave Macmillan.

Gondolf, Edward W. 2002. *Batterer intervention systems: Issues, outcomes, and recommendations, Sage Series on Violence Against Women*. London: Sage Publications.

Langeland, Eva, A.K. Wahl, K. Kristoffersen, and B.R. Hanestad. 2007. 'Promoting coping: Salutogenesis among people with mental health problems.' *Issues in Mental Health Nursing* 28 (3):275–295.

Sadler, J.Z. 2005. *Values and psychiatric diagnosis*. Oxford: Oxford University Press.

Yoder, Scot D. 2002. 'Individual responsibility for health: Decision, not discovery.' *Hastings Center Report* 32 (2):22–31.

7 *Sense of safety whole person domains* – mapping how much of Humpty we need to consider

- Aspects of the person that are impacted by threat and safety include: environment, social climate, relationships, body, experience, sense of self and meaning and spirit
- These are mapped as the *sense of safety whole person domains*
- An adequate breadth of inquiry prevents spurious precision

How much of Humpty do we need to consider? If we have a diagnosis that fits with the current paradigm of healthcare, is that enough, or is there a wider view required for those who encounter complexity and are oriented toward healing?

A colleague once described a teenager from a remote part of Australia who had presented saying he couldn't wear shorts in summer because his legs were too hairy. The practitioner examined his legs a number of times and didn't see the reported hairiness. After discussion with a psychiatrist, the teenager was diagnosed with 'body dysmorphic disorder' and trialled on some antidepressants. When these didn't have any impact, in desperation, a blood sample was sent by air to the city laboratory for new genetic testing that might reveal which antidepressant may be most effective. Even though the practitioner knew the wider story of this boy's life story, he became focussed on the lure of certainty in a technological genetic test or a neat psychiatric classification. This very isolated teen, experiencing peer bullying at school, whose father had left home as a child and whose stepfather had denied him access to a much-loved grandfather, was classified and tested. The complex relational reasons for his shaming critique of his body were largely ignored. Whole person healing is more relational, complex and ordinary and may take more time (at least in the short term) than writing a script or blood test form. Later discussion enlarged to what this practitioner could do to advocate for him at school and encourage the boy to reconnect with his grandfather. Keeping sight of the complex whole is a key generalist skill that requires reflection, collegiate discussion and a coherent mindset that can weigh up the integral value of each part of a wider whole.

Missing part of the whole is a daily experience for generalists. Sometimes it is a key piece of the puzzle – such as the importance of the diabetes experience of my patient's grandmother, as mentioned in Chapter Two. Sometimes it is a diagnosis that purports to explain a whole situation (such as 'body dysmorphic disorder' or 'social anxiety') that is so limited in what it has considered – for example, not attending to bullying, loneliness or shame – that its precision blinds the clinician to the whole. Sometimes it's a physical experience (such as pelvic pain) or an emotion (such as feeling trapped or hopeless) that is actually a flashback to past experiences in a patient's life story. They are memorial experiences triggered by the present. The accuracy of diagnosis is affected by how widely patient and practitioner look. Anything that is too narrow becomes spuriously precise (Wood, Allen, and Pantelis 2009).

A clinician on the frontline, dealing with undifferentiated distress, cannot deliver an exhaustive list of questions. An endless search for relevant information is not even possible in some research cohorts. The exhaustive breadth of scope is just not practical. So, the question for any generalist in any setting is how wide to look? How do we justify the breadth (what content areas do we consider?), length (how much past history is relevant?) and depth (how much insight is needed?) of information we seek to know before a diagnosis? These are practical questions, but they also are philosophical questions – what knowledge is important for meaningful generalist decision-making in any field? This question of the breadth of information also impacts research validity.

As outlined in earlier chapters, there is a philosophical need to include diverse forms of knowledge as part of a whole. Transdisciplinary literature supports the thesis that anything that causes a sense of threat is relevant to human wellbeing. There is also a need to consider the degree of threat and patterns that reveal threat, which will be discussed in later chapters. When considering whole person scope, objective physical and subjective causes of threat are both part of the whole. Seeing threat from a strengths-based approach means searching for resources that contribute to a *sense of safety*.

In my doctoral research, I therefore asked stakeholders two main questions:

What threatens people?
How do people sense that they are safe?

Stakeholder responses and discussions were analysed and themes of *content* and *process* were identified.[1] Process themes became known as *sense of safety dynamics*, discussed in the following chapters. Seven areas of content were identified as *sense of safety whole person domains* and were mapped.

The *sense of safety whole person domains* are presented as a map in Figure 7.1. This map could be used as a way to define the breadth of what might impact wellbeing – a kind of systems review for the practitioner. It could also be used by employers to map their employee services, or for schools to map whole person approaches to child behaviour and learning needs or for Humpty to understand himself. It may also be useful for wider health prioritising, policy decisions and service mapping.

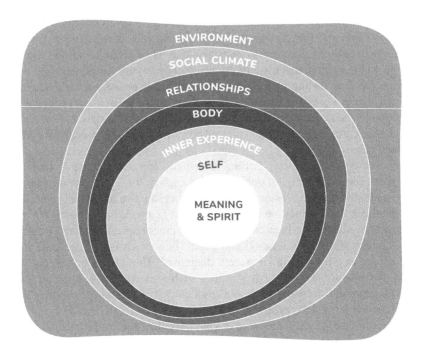

Figure 7.1 Sense of safety whole person domains.

Although named and often researched separately, these domains are part of a unified whole. They are integrated and interconnected within the person who is embedded within their relational and environmental context. There are intrapersonal, neural and meaningful connections between aspects of the person and intersubjective, interpersonal and sensory connection to others and the environment. A map that maintains a complex generalist awareness of the whole person could be useful if it was deemed a valid inclusive framework for decision-making. It would mean that even when a part is considered (e.g., thoughts of suicide, blood test results, work or school performance or research into a 'body part'), the whole would not be minimised or ignored. It would mean that even when a person feels and presents as fragmented or insistently focuses on one aspect of their distress, the practitioner has a way to maintain a stable intentional awareness of the coherent whole. This is whole person care in action.

Enlarging on the insight that a 'sense of safety' includes self, other and context, stakeholder responses to what causes threat and builds safety have revealed a framework that could help practitioners reflect systematically on the whole. In any consideration of the whole, the practitioner needs a breadth of awareness that considers the domains of: *environment, social climate, relationships, body, experience, sense of self* and *meaning and spirit*. Each of these whole person domains will be discussed below, as they emerged from stakeholder consultation. Transdisciplinary literature relevant to each domain will also be outlined. A table of summarised direct quotes of stakeholder feedback, including key quotes and a key question for practitioner reflection, is included for each domain. This documentation of stakeholder direct quotes of insights includes the breadth of negative and positive responses in each domain, maintaining the commitment to not narrowing attention too early and allowing practitioner readers to apply what is relevant to their own context.

Environment

This term was chosen (rather than 'context') to reflect the strong themes of the importance of country and climate to many stakeholders' *sense of safety*. Stakeholders mentioned physical environment, equity, stability, access and freedom in the experience of *sense of safety*. Waiting, vulnerability, unpredictability, isolation, racism, criminalisation, frightening or pessimistic news, change and unhelpful services were themes of threat to safety in the environment. The importance of connection to country was mentioned by GPs and indigenous academics. When prompted by the term 'context', GPs said they were aware of the seasons, drought, time of day or year and school environment. See Table 7.1. The domain of environment is therefore defined as 'awareness of physical environment, time, information and processes of equity or its absence in the political, financial, occupational, social and intellectual environment'.

The *environment* domain is mirrored in the literature that addresses social determinants of health (Marmot 2005, Wallace and Wallace 1997, Carson et al.

Table 7.1 Summary of *Environment Whole Person Domain*

Physical environment, time, information and processes of equity or its absence in the political, financial, occupational, social and intellectual environment
'it will either feel OK or not OK in that environment' (ia)
'safe place to sleep' (mhc)
'What has happened to you' (le)
Physical environment: connection to country, massacre places, drought, isolation, climate change, food and water security, war, darkness, housing, crowding, noise, childcare, medical setting, comfort of waiting room, needles, fulfilling basic needs, shelter, transport, global financial crisis, personal finances, workplace, protection from perpetrators
Time and information: 'giving us enough time to feel safe' (ia); diagnosis, pessimistic news or stories in the home or inadequate information: 'not knowing feels very unsafe' (gp)
Equity: politics, power, corruption, racism – 'more than neglect' (ia), affordability, availability, unequal division of resources, caring government and health system, reliable police, accessible health care, intellectual freedom, explanations, time valued, fear of being reported to government, democracy, unsupportive organisations, national and international instability, powerlessness, 're-traumatisation through government policies' (ia), access to meaningful occupation or self-development
Key question: Do you have anywhere to rest where you are not feeling threatened?

2007), living conditions such as housing security (Thurston et al. 2013), crowding and noise (Sayin et al. 2015) and psychological safety at work (Kark and Carmeli 2009). Water security, food security, equity and political, policing and international security affect 'human security' (Hughes and Rowe 2007, Buzan 2007, Gleick 1993, Pinstrup-Andersen 2009, Cook and Bakker 2012, Paris 2001, Browne et al. 2012). Processes of injustice, incarceration corruption, migration and racism impact safety and health (MacKenzie and Goodstein 1985, Chao et al. 2014, Levy and Sidel 2013, Tepper 2001, D'Monte 2000, Hofrichter 2003). Research into the health impact of a person's 'life world' is relevant to primary care (Todres, Galvin, and Dahlberg 2007, Barry et al. 2001). Climate change has also raised awareness of the impact of environment on wellbeing (Fritze et al. 2008, Zhang et al. 2018). Maslow named basic needs relevant to this domain: 'freedom to speak, freedom to express oneself, freedom to investigate and seek for information, freedom to defend oneself, justice, fairness, honesty and orderliness' (Maslow 1954, 22). A key aspect of this dynamic is order and justice (a form of social coherence). These freedoms in the environment are part of a *sense of safety* and contribute to integrity, connection and coherence and the aspect of the *sense of safety* framework called *safe place to be* (see Chapter Four).

Social climate

The importance of the social atmosphere at home, school and in the wider community and culture was made clear through stakeholder consultations. There is still substantial overlap with the domain of environment as these two domains are so interconnected (e.g., shelter or 'safe place to sleep' can be influenced by environmental and relational dynamics). The domain of *social climate* attends to the overall experience of *home* and social environment, places where *living and learning* happen and overall *culture and community* (including intergenerational impacts). Stakeholders mentioned the importance of culture, of intellectual freedom, respect and being connected to more than one person. One stakeholder spoke of the impact of frightening stories being told around children. Threats to *sense of safety* that were mentioned included lack of bridging language, social instability, being a minority, racism, being treated as worthless by a social group, alcoholism, homelessness, unpayable bills, fear of job loss, scary people, social media, generational trauma and threat or challenge to identity. GPs, when prompted with the term 'social climate' or 'context', said they also assessed past child rearing; how well they knew the patient; the degree of trust and understanding; dynamics of shared housing; access to learning, jobs, and healthcare and the degree of hope in their context. See Table 7.2. This domain is defined as 'awareness of the atmosphere at home, where you live and learn and in the wider community and culture (including intergenerational processes and social media)'.

Transdisciplinary literature confirms the impact of the social environment at home, work, school, wider community and culture on health. Experiences of hopelessness, workaholism, perfectionism, alcoholism, gambling, violence or volatility at home cause morbidity and mortality (Tziner and Tanami 2013,

Table 7.2 Summary of *Social Climate Whole Person Domain*

Atmosphere at home, where you live and learn, and in the wider community and culture (including intergenerational processes and social media)

'culture fundamentally is how a person relates to society' (gp)

'a safe place to sleep' (mhc)

Home: living situation, shelter, privacy, affordability, predictability or instability, not crowded, migration, where they've lived (including changes), remoteness, warmth, hope, transport, noise, cash flow, clothes, drugs and alcohol, alcoholism, intoxication, past child rearing, small spaces, loud voices, trapped, no escape, safe place to sleep, domestic violence, what you perceive to be normal, criminalisation, fear of police or child safety services, availability of financial back up

Live and learn: education environment, financial security, poverty, cash flow, job availability, work environment, pessimistic news, TV, radio, newspaper, diagnosis, illness, unfamiliar, fear of job loss, respected at work, 'your ability to access and act on those things' (gp)

Culture and community (including intergenerational processes): safe cultural practices, rules, rituals, stories, who talks?, proud of where you came from, family connections extending back, interactions in community, racism, trauma in previous generations, migration, belief systems, minority, language, respect for people's connection to country

Key question: Do you have a safe place to be in your community (including online)?

Robinson 1998, Griffiths et al. 2005, Anda et al. 2006). The absence of relationships in chronic fatherlessness, or parental absence through illness, incarceration or mental illness, or even dislocation from extended family are known causes of distress (Gelles 1989, Porter and Haslam 2005, Adams and Horovitz 1980).

Feeling safe at work impacts creativity, productivity, learning and self-expression (Kark and Carmeli 2009, Edmondson 2004). Unsafe workplaces are described as having VUCA – volatility, uncertainty, complexity, ambiguity (Bennett and Lemoine 2014). Organisational psychologists ask: 'what allows people to openly share ideas and contribute part of themselves to a collaborative undertaking?' (Edmondson 2004, 240), a question relevant to therapeutic relationships and to the safety of family or kinship groupings.

Cultural safety (Anderson et al. 2003) is also part of the social climate that people live in, including cultural experiences of community (Kilcullen, Swinbourne, and Cadet-James 2012) or cultural and transgenerational experiences of dispossession, migration, violation, oppression, socioeconomic disadvantage or disenfranchised loss (Faimberg 2005, Vivero and Jenkins 1999). Even the built environment research notes the importance of relational solidarity in a community impacting *sense of safety* (Kuo, Bacaicoa, and Sullivan 1998). Whether at home, where you live and learn, or in the wider community, a sense of being settled and belonging are key elements of this domain. They contribute to many aspects of *sense of safety* – creating a place where it is *safe to belong* and where it is *safe enough to grow.*

Relationships

This domain relates to personal relationships in the person's life. It attends to *who* is in the person's life, *what* that relationship is like (including lost relationship from many causes) and *how* that relationship is conducted (including tone of voice, trust, attunement and reliability). Stakeholders mentioned family, sexual relationships, friends, carers, neighbours, children, extended family and therapeutic relationships. Roles and family dynamics, loss and confrontation were all mentioned. Many threats to *sense of safety* from relationships were described. As mentioned in Chapter Five, the general themes of threat from how relationships were conducted included *disconnection, invasion* and *confusion*.

Experiences of safety in relationships seemed to be linked to belonging, trust, being heard and understood, a sense of meaningful support and being treated with dignity. Additional relationships that GPs said they already assessed included awareness of power dynamics and capacity to negotiate in past and present relationships. They also mentioned teachers, sporting teams, coaches, parents and the person's boss. This domain relates to personal connections and has some overlap with the domain of social climate. See Table 7.3. This domain is defined as 'awareness of who is in your environment, what interactions you have – including loss of relationships and how those relationships are conducted (including your physical reaction to them)'.

Literature confirms the importance of the 'social synapse' (Cozolino 2006, 6) or intersubjective space (Stolorow 2000) and the ways that humans co-regulate emotion (Butler and Randall 2013) in a 'shared bio-behavioural state' (Geller and Porges 2014, 185). The attachment and neurobiological literature confirms the importance of attuned responsive reliable relationships and their impact on physiology, including immunology, metabolism, neural connectivity and neural structures (in negative or positive neuroplasticity) (Schore 2001, Fagundes, Glaser, and Kiecolt-Glaser 2013, Tomasdottir et al. 2015), especially at key times in development and in intimate relationships (Gouin and Kiecolt-Glaser 2011). Research confirms the importance of interpersonal reflective function – mentalising, empathy, compassion, trust, social engagement and even love (Porges 2003, Allen 2013, Burnette et al. 2009, Endreß and Pabst 2013, Sbarra and Hazan 2008). The capacity to mentalise is a building block for maternal-infant responsiveness, coherent narratives, affect regulation and social connectedness (Allen 2013, Bateman and Fonagy 2012, Pajulo et al. 2012).

Loss of safe relationships is documented in the literature on disconnection, emotional and physical absence, loneliness (Hawkley and Cacioppo 2010), social withdrawal, social exclusion (Twenge, Catanese, and Baumeister 2003), social rejection (Slavich et al. 2010), social pain (Eisenberger et al. 2011), betrayal (Freyd, Klest, and Allard 2005) and bullying (Lereya et al. 2015). Trauma is defined as 'violation of an expectancy to be safe with another' (Porges 2014) and 'repeatedly being left psychologically alone in unbearable emotional pain' (Allen 2013, xxii), highlighting the central role of relationships and their impact on the self (Courtois and Ford 2009). The key theme of this domain is connection and

Table 7.3 Summary of *Relationship Whole Person Domain*

Who is in your environment, what interactions you have – including loss of relationships and how those relationships are conducted (including your physical reaction to them)

'honour, dignity, trustworthy, compassion in relationship' (le)
'accepted, nurtured, protected, encouraged' (mhc)
'feel held and whole' (gp)
'others to reach out to when overwhelmed' (mhc)
'be able to allow others to safely be who they are' (gp)

WHO is in your world?: family (parents, children, partner), romantic relationship, close friends, neighbours, coach, sporting team, boss, work, authority figures, community, professionals, receptionists, social media

WHAT interactions do you have? (including loss of relationship): supply of relationships, number in network, loss of relationship, divorce, custody, roles, family dynamics, intergenerational history, cyberbullying, domestic violence, crime, history of relationships, terror of touch, sexuality, racism, unexplained difference, expectations, past betrayals of trust, fear of incompetence, angry expressions, distance, change, uniforms, loneliness, confrontation, disharmony, not belonging, threat or actual loss of relationship, inability to care for offspring, feeling no one is 'with them', socialising, sharing experiences, expectations, personal freedom, financial freedom, 'able to express myself' (gp), understandable language

HOW are those relationships conducted?: tone of voice (e.g., sharp tone), welcome, accepted, warmth, rapport, support, alliance, stability, meaningful support, love from a care figure, attunement, respected, listened to, heard, not judged, kindness, trust, presence, spend time, honest, genuine, congruent, belonging, 'not too close or too far' (mhc), power dynamic, able to negotiate, 'intimacy and equality of relationships' (mhc), apologies, personal freedom in relationships, financial freedom, respect – don't have to 'tippy-toe around' (gp), startle reflex, reactions to uniforms, able to negotiate, 'respectful interaction' (gp), 'supported, attunement, empowered, collaborative therapeutic relationships – walk journey together' (gp), misunderstood, judged, controlling relationships, discounted, exploited, volatile, dehumanised, shamed, violated, blamed, bullied, marginalised, aggression, exposed, criticised, torture, disrespect, ignore, reject, invaded, disconnect, abandon, frighten, betray, restrict, trap, verbal/physical abuse, intimidation, exclusion, loneliness

Key question: In your closest relationships is there fun and safe warm connection?

---

affection as part of *sense of safety*, although integrity and coherence are also part of safe relationships, making it safe to belong.

Body

This domain includes stakeholder descriptions of their own or another person's physical being that are relevant for a *sense of safety* or threat. These included awareness of *physical body, movement and behaviour, awareness and sensation* and *capacity for regulation.* Stakeholders mentioned awareness of their own body and their capacity to perceive through their senses and respond to other people's physical presence. Stakeholders noticed appearance, body language, mobility and facial expressions. Sleep, diet, substance use, medications, exercise, hormones, emotion, temperature, heart rate, allergens, disease, physical distress, mobility and ageing were also mentioned. Stakeholders discussed the influence of genetics, personality, temperament and sensitivity to stimuli (including touch and needles). Key bodily experiences that stakeholders felt were threatening included arousal, intoxication, shame, hunger, pain, foreboding, hypervigilance, flooding emotions and anxiety. Stakeholders also raised concerns about the physical impact of a lifetime of extreme stress, violence and fight/flight reactions. The inner experience of illness or cancer as loss of control was described as 'threat from within' (mhc). The fear 'do we have something wrong with us?' was also named. Additional aspects that GPs mentioned when prompted about the body were red flags of cancer, family history of illness, lifestyles, sexual activity and contraception, past torture, the capacity to experience touch and 'physical safety from a medical perspective, because that is what they're seeing you for' (gp). See Table 7.4. This domain is defined as awareness of 'physical body, movement and behaviour, awareness, sensation and regulation'.

Table 7.4 Summary of *Body Whole Person Domain*

Physical body, movement and behaviour, awareness, sensation and regulation

'sense bodily calm' (mhc)
'the body holds everything' (ia)
'dealing with body respectfully' (gp)

Physical body: integrity, calm, death, illness 'threat from within' (mhc), body habitus, racing heart, acute/chronic, nutrition, family history, fight/flight, exposed, life time of extreme stress, 'cancer inside you' (gp), red flags, anaemia, ageing, infection, allergens, 'drugs that are cruel to the body' (le)

Movement and behaviour: appropriate touch, permission, consent, body language, tone of voice, dress, facial expressions, gait, sexual activity, family lifestyle, exercise, dance, sing, rituals, aggression, sexualised behaviour (in children), mobility, strong reaction to PAP smear [gynaecological examination], startle reflex, 'seeing how the person presents themselves and relates to you' (gp), 'feel unsafe and react to that without having necessarily that high level of cognition able to recognise "I'm not feeling safe and that is why I'm reacting this way"' (gp)

Awareness and sensation (including arousal, intuition, consciousness): vision and other senses, sounds, smells, presence, hunger, pain, intense emotion, concentration, perception, shame, foreboding, tense, nausea, hypervigilance, 'overwhelming can't' (ia), 'arousal prevents safety' (mhc), 'take it in through all their senses, some of which they may not be consciously aware of and it they're not … then they filter it through the maps in their mind' (gp), disorientation, tiredness, 'understanding what is happening?' (le), subconscious, 'conscious enough that they know where it is that decision is going to take them'(gp)

Regulation: drugs and alcohol, sleep, appetite, self-medicating, intoxication, flooding, overwhelm, bodily calm, hormones, temperature, heart rate, blood pressure, 'parasympathetic state if supported and safe' (gp), 'they need to learn to contain' (gp)
Key question: Can you help your body to feel calm for moments of your day?

Transdisciplinary literature confirms the importance of the body's response to our life story with experiences 'inscribed on all bodily levels (organs, tissues, cells and genes)' (Kirkengen and Thornquist 2012). The body is impacted by interpersonal, intrapersonal and memorial experiences, whether 'perceived, experienced or reactivated' (Kirkengen and Thornquist 2012, 1470). As mentioned in Chapter Five, the body interacts with the person's world – nociception and 'neuroception' of danger – through the five senses, proprioception and interoception (Ogden, Minton, and Pain 2006). The immune system is also a sensory system that responds to internal threats (Blalock 1984, Dantzer et al. 2008) and links directly with the autonomic nervous system (Elenkov et al. 2000). The body enacts dynamic responses to the physical and social environment and circadian and energy demands. Biomarkers of stress, including cortisol levels and heart rate variability are increasingly being understood as ways to understand physical illness (Beauchaine 2015). The body can also reveal threat through posture, prosody (tone of voice), movement, scars, self-harming behaviours, pain, obsessions, startle reaction and agitation.

Research into multimorbidity and allostatic load as mentioned earlier also confirm the impact of loss of safety on the body through 'multisystem physiological dysregulation' (Wiley et al. 2016). This 'weathering' (Geronimus et al. 2006) includes altered glucocorticoid regulation, immune and endocrine responses (Lupien et al. 2009, Gutteling, de Weerth, and Buitelaar 2005, Juster, McEwen, and Lupien 2010). Traumatic experiences also cause loss of synaptic connectivity and neuronal survival (Perry et al. 1995), including loss of corpus callosum interhemispheric connectivity (Teicher et al. 2016) and many other structural brain changes. These 'experience-based anatomical changes in brain structure' (Scaer 2014, 61) can affect access to language, reason, affect regulation and approach valence, producing changes that are adaptive in threatening environments, but maladaptive once away from danger (Teicher et al. 2016).

An overall 'visceral sense of control and safety', as described by Bessel van der Kolk (2014, 31), is a way to describe the physicality of a *sense of safety*. Other aspects of the physical body that are relevant in a whole person assessment include appearance, physiology, emotion, memory, sensation, arousal and behaviour. Table 7.5 reminds us of the importance of these aspects of the dynamic sensory conscious body – including the physical nature of emotion and memory. The key theme of this domain is a settled, calm, aware body – part of the overarching process of *calm body* and being *safe on the inside*. This includes bodily *integrity*, regulation at multiple levels (*coherence*) and being embedded in safe relationships (*connection*).

Inner experience

This domain intentionally attends to any descriptions of the subjective inner world of the person that stakeholders mentioned or alluded to. Words associated with this domain are present in other domains and are often implied in language around memory, emotion, thoughts, attention, perception, understanding and connection.

Table 7.5 Aspects of the Body That Are Part of Sensing Safety of the Whole

Aspect of the body	Aspects for clinician to attend to
Appearance	Subtle changes in prosody (Grandjean et al. 2005), facial expressions, startle reflex, response to touch, body language, dress, hygiene, physical illness, pain and injury
Physiology	Nutritional, cardiac, respiratory, metabolic, immunologic and endocrine factors that influence the whole person and can be influenced by stress (Anisman and Zacharko 1990)
Emotions	Understood as meaningful physical responses to threat and safety in the environment (Matthieu and Ivanoff 2006) – 'a kind of perception of our own bodily state' (Blazer 2005, 188) ... 'hard-wired neural circuits in the visceral-limbic brain that facilitate diverse and adaptive behavioural and physiological responses' (Panksepp 1982, 407) Emotion reveals subjective experience and is expressed in behavioural and biological markers
Memory	Implicit and explicit verbal memory (Schacter, Bowers, and Booker 1989), aware of dissociative amnesia in response to fear or overwhelm, embodied memories re-experienced as flashbacks and autobiographical coherence (Siegel 2001, Siegel 2010)
Sensation	The eight senses, including sight, sound, touch, taste, smell, proprioception, vestibular sensation and interoception (Critchley et al. 2004) and capacity to attend to sensation (Barrett et al. 2004) Sensation can be affected by stress and avoidance of previous overwhelming sensations (Van der Kolk and McFarlane 2012)
Arousal	Note altered awareness of time, capacity for coherent narrative, embodiment, awareness of affect (including alexithymia) and interpersonal experience of another person (Thompson and Zahavi 2007) – trauma related altered states of consciousness (Frewen et al. 2015)
Behaviour	Awareness of the degree of organised, regulated rhythmic behaviour and watching for dysregulation, disorganisation or incoherent behaviour, including changes in avoidance (Koopman et al. 2003) or approach behaviours (Harmon-Jones and Allen 1998) This includes awareness of ambivalence, obsessions, cravings, addictive coping styles and reward seeking behaviour. Loss of routine (e.g., sleep, diet), normal desires (e.g., libido and motivation), restorative processes (e.g., rest and relaxation), movement, engagement in meaningful occupation, creativity and adaptation to change

Stakeholders also gave an insight into the range of experiences, including distortions, confusions, fears and compulsions (as well as peace, order, comfort and connection), that impact *sense of safety*. Inner experiences stakeholders mentioned that threaten *sense of safety* were shame, uncertainty, unknowing, intense emotion, fear, avoidance, pain, vulnerability, exposure, loss of control, hopelessness and powerlessness. The name 'inner experience' for this domain came after GPs described a need to differentiate inner subjective experience from external events that are often,

Table 7.6 Summary of *Inner Experience Whole Person Domain*

Thoughts, attention, memories, perceptions, senses, intuition, mood states and self-talk

'compute inside myself'
'feel safe with capacity' (mhc)
'still themselves and allow whatever thoughts that were rubbing around to flow through them' (ia)
'perceptions and assumptions may be wildly inaccurate' (gp)
'feeling of unsafeness from their past gets triggered in current life situations' (mhc)

Includes: thoughts, memories, mood states, interpretations, perceptions, assumptions, senses, unconscious, intuition, instinct, self-talk, triggers, decisions, attention

Peace/comfort: 'able to relax, reduce monitoring my environment' (mhc), good decisions, calmness, 'being able to think clearly and creatively' (mhc), more comfortable with GPs they have known for a while, sense of freedom, 'own their mind' (gp), self-esteem, confidence in self, integrity – personal and professional

Connected: heard, validated, present, 'space for the unspeakable to be spoken' (ia)

Organise: 'compute inside myself' (ia), 'unsafe or feel safe to connect to this relationship' (ia), 'actually name feelings that are flooding within' (ia), story from your point of view, remember my past, 'filter sense through maps in their mind which is based on their past experience ... then put it all together. Most of that is unconscious. If you ask them they will just know they feel safe or unsafe' (gp), 'titrate with them up and down' (ia), grief

Confusion: ambivalence, uncertainty, fear of unknown, misunderstood, no idea why, what's behind your body language, paranoia, hopelessness, unable to read another person, incongruences in the story, 'lose boundaries of the edge of themselves' (gp), tension between thinking and feeling brain

Shame: dealing with shame and embarrassment, feeling blamed, unable to express openly, vulnerable, judged, feeling unable to meet expectations, weak self-efficacy, failure, insecure

Invasion: self-harm, challenged, anger, pressures, expectations, intimidated, invalidation

Disconnection: not listened to, avoidant, no curiosity, isolation, dishonesty, excluded, not belonging

Out of control: no control, powerlessness, frustrated, pain, discomfort, depression, injustice, constrained, loss, emotional overload

Fear: 'constant fear' (gp), anxiety, trapped, dependant, 'experience the world as exceptionally unsafe' (mhc)

Key question: Can you find comfort to still your mind and see things in perspective calmly?

---

named 'experiences' by those who see the world through a positivist objective lens. See Table 7.6. The domain of *inner experience* is defined as 'thoughts, attention, memories, perceptions, senses, intuition, mood states and self-talk'.

The literature on attention, effortful control, cognitions, self-talk and emotion regulation is especially relevant to this domain (Bögels and Mansell 2004, Crombez et al. 1999, Lavie, Beck, and Konstantinou 2014, Rothbart and Rueda 2005, Preece et al. 2018). Emotional thought (Immordino Yang and Damasio 2007) and cognitions can be suppressed (Borkovec and Lyonfields 1993), intrusive (Kent et al. 2000), ruminating (Watkins 2008), ambivalent, incoherent, rigid and automatic or creative, reflective, insightful and mindful (Dietrich and Haider 2017, Sugarman 2006, Tuch 2007). Threat and safety can be experienced internally causing a long-term inner atmosphere that impacts health (Gilbert 1993). Literature on inner dialogue is extensive and will be considered in more detail in the domain of *sense of self* and the dynamic of *respectful connection* in Chapter Nine. Again, an experience of an internal sense of integrity, connection, and coherence contributes to the overarching theme of safe on the inside.

Sense of self

This domain captures communication and attitudes (or relationship) towards the self. Safety was a theme of inner respectful connecting relationship –contributing to *dignity*, *trust* and *unity* that could also be understood as integrity, connection and coherence. Inner attitudes of respect, integrity, trust of self, connection with self, acceptance, worthiness, stability, confidence and feeling loved were mentioned as part of a *sense of safety*. Understanding and listening to inner dialogue was also mentioned. Negative inner dialogue about worth, and belonging were mentioned as threats to *sense of safety* – such as 'you're not good enough', 'you don't belong' and 'who do you think you are' (ia). Loss of confidence, shame, invalidation, loss of trust in self and attacks on reputation were also mentioned. As one GP stated: 'It's not safe if you don't like yourself' (gp). Additional aspects that GPs mentioned that they already assessed in this area included 'how they are feeling about themselves in the world' (gp), how they see themselves, 'what they are good at' (gp) and observations of facial expressions, engagement, humour and conversational skills. See Table 7.7. The domain of *sense of self* is defined as 'inner connection and communication towards the self that impacts dignity and trust and inner unity'.

Although the concept of 'self' is contested, a neurobiological understanding of the term may be useful in this context: 'the self is a construction of its relation with itself' (Kircher and David 2003, 1). Meares notes the sensorimotor, meaningful (semantic) and reflective tiers of the self linked to the development of memory that cooperate and coordinate to form the self (Meares 2019). The literature on self-awareness, identity (Stamenov 2003, 81), self-efficacy, self-compassion (Leary et al. 2007) and self-regulation (Ford et al. 2005) are relevant to this domain. Key primary care researchers have identified a GP role in enabling and restoring sense of self (Reeve 2010, Stone 2013, Dowrick 2004, Dowrick et al. 2016, Dowrick 2017). Grief researchers describe working towards a 'multifaceted, dynamic and narrative' self (Neimeyer 2001, 216) or 'reconstituting the self' (Neimeyer 2001, 213).

The literature on voice hearing as 'altered self-awareness' (Henriksen, Raballo, and Parnas 2015, 189) or 'estrangement' (Stamenov 2003, 76) from self, reveals a loss of inner trust, unity and self-respect in line with the findings from stakeholder consultation. Objectifying and shaming the self is inherently threatening. This can occur due to inner disunity or ambivalence among parts of the self or inner disgust, self-loathing (Dorahy et al. 2015) (Nathanson 1994, Gruenewald et al. 2004), self-criticism (Priel and Shahar 2000, Shahar et al. 2012) or other forms of

Table 7.7 Summary of *Sense of Self Whole Person Domain*

Inner connection and communication towards self that impacts dignity and trust and inner unity
'inner thoughts about yourself' (le) **'it's not safe if you don't like yourself' (gp)** **'I'm strong in my identity, I'm loved, and I'm surrounded by what I choose in my environment' (ia)**

Inner attitudes and communication towards self:
Relationship with self (gp), who am I?
Dignity: self-worth, self-respect, feeling good enough, valid, worthy, identity, 'it's about your entitlement to being on the planet and sucking up oxygen' (gp), 'sense that they are accepted and they matter' (mhc), respect, reputation, valid
Trust of self: 'own myself and my experiences' (le), 'OK to make mistakes' (gp), 'vital to our wellbeing that we get to know/listen and understand our inner dialogue' (le), vulnerable, 'it's very important for a person to feel safe within themselves' (gp)
Unified self: 'way of being themselves isn't their whole self' (gp), 'a little voice inside your heart that says you are not good enough' (ia), 'inner berating' (ia), 'broken down' (gp)
Key question: Are you feeling safe enough in yourself to face this challenge?

empathic failure towards the self (Neimeyer and Jordan 2002). As Louis Cozolino (2006, 316) says: 'love is a relief from scanning the outer world for threat and the inner world for shame'.

Trauma researchers suggest that therapeutic clinicians need an 'understanding of the nature of the divided self' (Phillips and Frederick 1995, 1) and warn that 'one of the robust findings in the neuroscience of early abuse and neglect is that kids who have to manage their feelings all by themselves learn to exclude their inner experiences from self-awareness and hence are prevented from developing such a robust sense of self' (Frewen and Lanius 2015, xvii). In fact, trauma researchers warn against simplistic views of the whole person as a unit – reminding clinicians to be aware of multiple 'states of consciousness' that one person can experience (Kezelman and Stavropoulos 2019). This complex view of the self as a whole made up of many parts raises awareness of the inner ambivalence and conflict that impact sense of capacity to cope with threat.

GP researchers note:

> Sense of self can be severely affected by the suffering they experience, whether the vitiating impact of socioeconomic deprivation, the fragmenting effects of sustained domestic violence, the catastrophic consequences of serious disease – or simply the effect of an imbalance between everyday demands and their resources to manage.
>
> (Dowrick et al. 2016, 582)

This domain has a theme of stability and inner unity (coherence), dignity (integrity) and inner trust or affection (connection) that contribute to being safe on the inside.

Meaning and spirit

This domain captures both a sense of personal meaning and fulfilment and any spiritual, religious or existential beliefs or concerns. Overall themes included *hope and purpose, sense-making, experience* and *connection.* Stakeholders described a sense of knowing 'who and why you are' (gp) and having 'something/one to lean on (God)' (mch), as well as a sense of purpose and hope. They named a capacity to explore or 'create your own meaning about your life story' (gp) as well as a sense of transcendence in soul or spirit, culture and country. Loss of hope, existential loss of security, shame, loss of faith, fear about the future and disrespect from others about your own beliefs were threats mentioned by stakeholders. Additional aspects that GPs mentioned that they already assessed included asking about religion and inner beliefs and also being aware of what the person is not saying, the sense of 'energy' about that person and 'being aware of what I may be missing' (gp). See Table 7.8. The domain of *meaning and spirit* is defined as 'experience of hope and purpose and connection and sense-making in cultural, religious or spiritual values and beliefs'.

Carey and Pilgrim (2010, 450) remind us that 'the nature and content of a person's distress is meaningful'. Maslow (1954, 5) affirms this – 'symptoms are important not so much in themselves, but for what they ultimately mean'. Sampson (1992, 512) adds, 'a person's beliefs about his reality are a central, organizing factor in his mental life, and such beliefs underlie maladaptation and psychopathology'. Isaac (2016, 1065) speaks of spirituality as an 'aspect of cultural identity that has become increasingly recognised for its potential to impact health behaviours and healthcare decision making'.

This domain also seeks to address the 'religiosity gap' between Humpty and those who care for him (Sperry 2002, Dein 2018). It enfranchises a way of knowing that is valued in transdisciplinary knowledge but which may be ignored if only positivist ways of knowing are valued. It includes the literature on the link between quality of life and spiritual needs (Lucchetti, Bassi, and Lucchetti 2013) and those who see it as part of multicultural whole person medicine (Anandarajah 2008). It aligns with Victor Frankl, an Auschwitz survivor, who states: 'healing comes from the realm of the spirit' (Frankl 1978, 23). The literature on meaning-making as a way to reconstruct order after loss (Neimeyer 2001), the existential elements of the post traumatic growth literature (Calhoun and Tedeschi 2006) and the focus on values in Acceptance Commitment Therapy (Harris 2006) and Logotherapy (Frankl 2014) are also relevant to this domain. This domain responds to the plea from experienced psychotherapist Karl Jung:

> But what will the doctor do when he sees only too clearly why his patient is ill; when he sees that it arises from his having no love, but only sexuality; no faith, because he is afraid to grope in the dark; no understanding, because he has failed to read the meaning of his own existence
>
> (Jung 1933, 225)

Table 7.8 Summary of *Meaning and Spirit Whole Person Domain*

Experience of hope and purpose, connection and sense-making in cultural, religious or spiritual values and beliefs

'I'm here for a reason ... faith that transcends life's circumstances' (mhc)
'where you came from, where you are going' (gp)
'you're trying to find the new meaning with change of circumstances, and that's sometimes difficult for people to find a safe place to do that' (gp)
'sense of hope ... turns perspective around' (gp)

Relevant areas: spiritual history, religion, meaning (including to be a patient), culture, beliefs, transcendence, values, inner beliefs, influence of family belief systems, connection to country, impact of other people and institutions on your meaning, cultural, family and contextual understandings

Hope and purpose: sense of purpose, loss of hope, meaningful contribution, 'meaningful work or creativity' (gp), 'sense of hope – turns perspective around' (gp), hopelessness

Sense-making: know who/why you are, where you came from/where you are going, 'existential loss of security (can be affected by the news)' (mhc), listen for meaning, 'here for a reason – transcends life's circumstances' (mhc), 'your self-understanding to create your own meaning about your own life' (gp), 'meaningful work or creativity' (gp)

Experience: spirituality, 'religious belief – spiritual fulfillment' (gp), 'their spirit is full of shame – their soul/spirit' (ia), fearful of punishment, 'some religions can create fear and you don't feel safe because you never know when someone's going to punish you spiritually' (gp), challenge to my religious belief (gp), 'seen as human ... respected as unique human being' (ia), loss of faith

Connected: 'acceptance of your world views, your village's views' (le), religion, 'sacred circle' (le)

Key question: Do you have any meaningful way to hold onto hope in the midst of your world?

Spirituality and organised communal ways of approaching these sense-making tasks such as religion, philosophy or culture can provide order (Mount 1993), context, peace and even transcendent attachment relationships (Kimball et al. 2013, Laurin, Schumann, and Holmes 2014) that can be experienced as comforting, hope giving and reconciling. The grief and loss literature also confirms that threat can also be experienced towards a person's worldview and beliefs or values; their prior assumptions can be shattered (Janoff-Bulman 1985), disconnected or disorganised. Indigenous lore is also seen as a way to order life meaningfully (Atkinson 2002). Life can also be experienced as meaningless (Newcomb and Harlow 1986) or hopeless (Anda et al. 1993), impacting wellbeing. This domain has an overarching theme of meaningful peace and hope, perhaps even purpose. Again, a sense of integrity to be free to believe, connection to belong to spiritual communities or forms of spirituality and the coherence of aligning with one's own values all contribute to being safe on the inside, experiencing a *safe place to be* and being *safe to belong*.

Each of these domains, as they have been described by stakeholders respond-ing to questions about safety and threat, include rich descriptions that could guide clinical awareness and prioritise care around safety and the whole person's experi-ence of self, other and context. This chapter has only touched on the relevant trans-disciplinary literature appropriate to each *sense of safety whole person domain*, and points towards a need for further intentional research (or simply collating current research) to explore the transdisciplinary relevance of breadth of content appraised to sense safety. These domains are the foundation of a coherent map of the whole person from the standpoint of the physiological and relational impact of threat. They map the breadth of content to search – revealing resources and protecting against threats in order to build a *sense of safety*. They are a transdis-ciplinary way of seeing the whole, built around trauma-informed, strengths-based and physiologically grounded evidence. Seeing and caring for the whole matters. They offer a shared language to define the breadth and types of knowing that is part of the endeavour to protect integrity, connection and coherence in any setting in the community.

Note

1 This thematic analysis is based on transcriptions of recordings of interviews and focus groups, post-it notes and white board memos. Most data included in this chap-ter emerged from open questions about what causes threat and how safety is sensed. Responses were sorted into those relevant to: "what helps people feel safe?" "what causes threat?" "what areas of a person's life is it important to feel safe in?" and "what do GPs already assess, or what do stakeholders add after domains are revealed?" Any conversations that occurred after the *sense of safety* concept and its domains were revealed (e.g., GPs' written responses to an additional question "what do you already assess?") were considered (and documented separately) in light of the fact that their responses were not de novo. Responses that referred to both resources for safety and potential for threat were included in this analysis. All responses relevant to breadth of appraisal were collated and coded. Relevant quotations are carefully recorded and coded into themes, which later became known as domains.

References

Adams, Paul L., and Jeffrey H. Horovitz. 1980. 'Psychopathology and fatherlessness in poor boys.' *Child Psychiatry and Human Development* 10 (3):135–143.

Allen, J.G. 2013. *Restoring mentalizing in attachment relationships: Treating trauma with plain old therapy*. Washington: American Psychiatric Publishing.

Anandarajah, Gowri. 2008. 'The 3 H and BMSEST models for spirituality in multicultural whole-person medicine.' *The Annals of Family Medicine* 6 (5):448–458.

Anda, R., V. Felitti, J. Bremner, J. Walker, Ch Whitfield, B. Perry, Sh Dube, and W. Giles. 2006. 'The enduring effects of abuse and related adverse experiences in childhood.' *European Archives of Psychiatry and Clinical Neuroscience* 256 (3):174–186. doi:10.1007/s00406-005-0624-4.

Anda, R., D. Williamson, D. Jones, C. Macera, E. Eaker, A. Glassman, and J. Marks. 1993. 'Depressed affect, hopelessness, and the risk of ischemic heart disease in a cohort of US adults.' *Epidemiology* 4 (4):285–294.

Anderson, Joan, Jo Ann Perry, Connie Blue, Annette Browne, Angela Henderson, Koushambhi Basu Khan, Sheryl Reimer Kirkham, Judith Lynam, Pat Semeniuk, and Vicki Smye. 2003. '"Rewriting" cultural safety within the postcolonial and postnational feminist project: Toward new epistemologies of healing.' *Advances in Nursing Science* 26 (3):196–214.

Anisman, Hymie, and Robert M. Zacharko. 1990. 'Multiple neurochemical and behavioral consequences of stressors: Implications for depression.' *Pharmacology & Therapeutics* 46 (1):119–136.

Atkinson, J. 2002. *Trauma trails: Recreating songlines. The transgenerational effects of trauma in Indigenous Australia.* Melbourne: Spinifex Press.

Barrett, Lisa Feldman, Karen S. Quigley, Eliza Bliss-Moreau, and Keith R. Aronson. 2004. 'Interoceptive sensitivity and self-reports of emotional experience.' *Journal of Personality and Social Psychology* 87 (5):684–697. doi:10.1037/0022-3514.87.5.684.

Barry, C.A., F.A. Stevenson, N. Britten, N. Barber, and C.P. Bradley. 2001. 'Giving voice to the lifeworld. More humane, more effective medical care? A qualitative study of doctor–patient communication in general practice.' *Social Science & Medicine* 53 (4):487–505.

Bateman, Anthony W., and Peter Fonagy. 2012. *Handbook of mentalizing in mental health practice.* Washington: American Psychiatric Publishing.

Beauchaine, Theodore P. 2015. 'Respiratory sinus arrhythmia: A transdiagnostic biomarker of emotion dysregulation and psychopathology.' *Current Opinion in Psychology* 3:43–47.

Bennett, Nathan, and G. James Lemoine. 2014. 'What a difference a word makes: Understanding threats to performance in a VUCA world.' *Business Horizons* 57 (3):311–317.

Blalock, Jeffrey Edwin. 1984. 'The immune system as a sensory organ.' *The Journal of Immunology* 132 (3):1067–1070.

Blazer, Dan German. 2005. *The age of melancholy: 'Major depression' and its social origins.* New York: Routledge.

Bögels, Susan M., and Warren Mansell. 2004. 'Attention processes in the maintenance and treatment of social phobia: Hypervigilance, avoidance and self-focused attention.' *Clinical Psychology Review* 24 (7):827–856.

Borkovec, Thomas D., and James D. Lyonfields. 1993. 'Worry: Thought suppression of emotional processing.' In *Attention and avoidance: Strategies in coping with aversiveness*, edited by H.W. Krohne, 101–118. Ashland, OH: Hogrefe & Huber Publishers.

Browne, Annette J., Colleen M. Varcoe, Sabrina T. Wong, Victoria L. Smye, Josée Lavoie, Doreen Littlejohn, David Tu, Olive Godwin, Murry Krause, and Koushambhi B. Khan. 2012. 'Closing the health equity gap: Evidence-based strategies for primary health care organizations.' *International Journal for Equity in Health* 11 (1):1–15.

Burnette, Jeni L., Don E. Davis, Jeffrey D. Green, Everett L. Worthington, and Erin Bradfield. 2009. 'Insecure attachment and depressive symptoms: The mediating role of rumination, empathy, and forgiveness.' *Personality and Individual Differences* 46 (3):276–280.

Butler, Emily A., and Ashley K. Randall. 2013. 'Emotional coregulation in close relationships.' *Emotion Review* 5 (2):202–210.

Buzan, Barry. 2007. *People, states and fear: An agenda for international security studies in the post-Cold War era, ECPR Classics (2nd).* Colchester: ECPR Press.

Calhoun, L.G., and R.G. Tedeschi, eds. 2006. *Handbook of posttraumatic growth. Research and practice*. Mahwah, NJ: Lawrence Erlbaum Associates.

Carey, Timothy A., and David Pilgrim. 2010. 'Diagnosis and formulation: What should we tell the students?' *Clinical Psychology & Psychotherapy* 17 (6):447–454.

Carson, Bronwyn, Terry Dunbar, Richard D. Chenhall, and Ross Bailie. 2007. *Social determinants of Indigenous health*. Crows Nest: Allen & Unwin.

Chao, Ruth Chu-Lien, Joseph Longo, Canzi Wang, Deepta Dasgupta, and Jessica Fear. 2014. 'Perceived racism as moderator between self-esteem/shyness and psychological distress among African Americans.' *Journal of Counseling & Development* 92 (3):259–269.

Cook, Christina, and Karen Bakker. 2012. 'Water security: Debating an emerging paradigm.' *Global Environmental Change* 22 (1):94–102.

Courtois, C., and Julian Ford, eds. 2009. *Treating complex Traumatic stress. An evidence based guide*. New York: The Guilford Press.

Cozolino, Louis, ed. 2006. *The neuroscience of human relationships. Attachment and the developing social brain*. New York: W.W. Norton and Company.

Critchley, Hugo D., Stefan Wiens, Pia Rotshtein, Arne Öhman, and Raymond J. Dolan. 2004. 'Neural systems supporting interoceptive awareness.' *Nature Neuroscience* 7 (2):189–195.

Crombez, Geert, Chris Eccleston, Frank Baeyens, Boudewijn Van Houdenhove, and Annelies Van Den Broeck. 1999. 'Attention to chronic pain is dependent upon pain-related fear.' *Journal of Psychosomatic Research* 47 (5):403–410.

Dantzer, Robert, Jason C. O'Connor, Gregory G. Freund, Rodney W. Johnson, and Keith W. Kelley. 2008. 'From inflammation to sickness and depression: When the immune system subjugates the brain.' *Nature Reviews Neuroscience* 9:46–56. https://doi.org/10.1038/nrn2297.

Dein, Simon. 2018. 'Against the stream: Religion and mental health–the case for the inclusion of religion and spirituality into psychiatric care.' *BJPsych Bulletin* 42 (3):127–129.

Dietrich, Arne, and Hilde Haider. 2017. 'A neurocognitive framework for human creative thought.' *Frontiers in Psychology* 7 (2078). doi:10.3389/fpsyg.2016.02078.

D'Monte, Darryl. 2000. 'Corruption, safety and environmental hazard in Asian societies.' *Economic and Political Weekly* 35 (33):2959–2968.

Dorahy, Martin J, Warwick Middleton, Lenaire Seager, Patrick McGurrin, Mary Williams, and Ron Chambers. 2015. 'Dissociation, shame, complex PTSD, child maltreatment and intimate relationship self-concept in dissociative disorder, chronic PTSD and mixed psychiatric groups.' *Journal of Affective Disorders* 172:195–203.

Dowrick, Christopher. 2004. *Beyond depression: A new approach to understanding and management*. London: Oxford University Press.

Dowrick, Christopher. 2017. *Person-centred primary care: Searching for the self*. London: Routledge.

Dowrick, Christopher, Iona Heath, Stefan Hjörleifsson, David Misselbrook, Carl May, Joanne Reeve, Deborah Swinglehurst, and Peter Toon. 2016. 'Recovering the self: A manifesto for primary care.' *British Journal of General Practice* 66 (652):582–583.

Edmondson, Amy. 2004. 'Psychological safety, trust and learning in organisation: A group-level lens.' In *Trust and distrust in organisations: Dilemmas and approaches*, edited by R.M. Kramer, and K.S. Cook, 239–272. New York: Russell Sage Foundation.

Eisenberger, N.I., S.L. Master, and T.K. Inagaki. 2011. 'Attachment figures activate a safety signal-related neural region and reduce pain experience.' *Proceedings of the National Academy of Sciences* 108 (28):11721–11726.

Elenkov, Ilia J., Ronald L. Wilder, George P. Chrousos, and E. Sylvester Vizi. 2000. 'The sympathetic nerve – an integrative interface between two supersystems: The brain and the immune system.' *Pharmacological Reviews* 52 (4):595–638.

Endreß, Martin, and Andrea Pabst. 2013. 'Violence and shattered trust: Sociological considerations.' *Human Studies* 36 (1):89–106.

Fagundes, Christopher P., Ronald Glaser, and Janice K. Kiecolt-Glaser. 2013. 'Stressful early life experiences and immune dysregulation across the lifespan.' *Brain, Behavior, and Immunity* 27:8–12.

Faimberg, Haydée. 2005. *The telescoping of generations: Listening to the narcissistic links between generations.* Hove: Routledge.

Ford, J.D., C.A. Courtois, K. Steele, O. Hart, and E.R.S. Nijenhuis. 2005. 'Treatment of complex posttraumatic self-dysregulation.' *Journal of Traumatic Stress* 18 (5):437–447.

Frankl, Viktor E. 1978. *The unheard cry for meaning: Psychotherapy and humanism.* Sydney: Hodder and Stoughton.

Frankl, Viktor E. 2014. *The will to meaning: Foundations and applications of logotherapy.* New York: Penguin.

Frewen, Paul, Kathy Hegadoren, Nick J. Coupland, Brian H. Rowe, Richard W.J. Neufeld, and Ruth Lanius. 2015. 'Trauma related altered states of consciousness (TRASC) and functional impairment 1: Prospective study in acutely traumatized persons.' *Journal of Trauma & Dissociation* 16 (5):500–519. doi:10.1080/1529973 2.2015.1022925.

Frewen, Paul, and Ruth Lanius. 2015. *Healing the traumatized self: Consciousness, neuroscience, treatment (Norton series on interpersonal neurobiology).* New York: W.W. Norton & Company.

Freyd, J.J., B. Klest, and C.B. Allard. 2005. 'Betrayal trauma: Relationship to physical health, psychological distress, and a written disclosure intervention.' *Journal of Trauma & Dissociation* 6 (3):83–104.

Fritze, Jessica G., Grant A. Blashki, Susie Burke, and John Wiseman. 2008. 'Hope, despair and transformation: Climate change and the promotion of mental health and wellbeing.' *International Journal of Mental Health Systems* 2 (13). https://doi.org/10.1186/1752 -4458-2-13.

Geller, Shari M., and Stephen W. Porges. 2014. 'Therapeutic presence: Neurophysiological mechanisms mediating feeling safe in therapeutic relationships.' *Journal of Psychotherapy Integration* 24 (3):178–192.

Gelles, Richard J. 1989. 'Child abuse and violence in single-parent families: Parent absence and economic deprivation.' *American Journal of Orthopsychiatry* 59 (4):492–501.

Geronimus, Arline T., Margaret Hicken, Danya Keene, and John Bound. 2006. '"Weathering" and age patterns of allostatic load scores among blacks and whites in the United States.' *American journal of Public Health* 96 (5):826–833.

Gilbert, Paul. 1993. 'Defence and safety: Their function in social behaviour and psychopathology.' *British Journal of Clinical Psychology* 32 (2):131–153.

Gleick, Peter H. 1993. 'Water and conflict: Fresh water resources and international security.' *International Security* 18 (1):79–112.

Gouin, Jean-Philippe, and Janice K. Kiecolt-Glaser. 2011. 'The impact of psychological stress on wound healing: Methods and mechanisms.' *Immunology and Allergy Clinics of North America* 31 (1):81–93.

Grandjean, Didier, David Sander, Gilles Pourtois, Sophie Schwartz, Mohamed L. Seghier, Klaus R. Scherer, and Patrik Vuilleumier. 2005. 'The voices of wrath: Brain responses to angry prosody in meaningless speech.' *Nature Neuroscience* 8 (2):145–146.

Griffiths, Mark, Adrian Parke, Richard Wood, and Jonathan Parke. 2005. 'Internet gambling: An overview of psychosocial impacts.' *UNLV Gaming Research & Review Journal* 10 (1):27–39.

Gruenewald, Tara L., Margaret E. Kemeny, Najib Aziz, and John L. Fahey. 2004. 'Acute threat to the social self: Shame, social self-esteem, and cortisol activity.' *Psychosomatic Medicine* 66 (6):915–924.

Gutteling, Barbara M., Carolina de Weerth, and Jan K. Buitelaar. 2005. 'Prenatal stress and children's cortisol reaction to the first day of school.' *Psychoneuroendocrinology* 30 (6):541–549.

Harmon-Jones, Eddie, and John J.B. Allen. 1998. 'Anger and frontal brain activity: EEG asymmetry consistent with approach motivation despite negative affective valence.' *Journal of Personality and Social Psychology* 74 (5):1310–1316.

Harris, Russell. 2006. 'Embracing your demons: An overview of acceptance and commitment therapy.' *Psychotherapy in Australia* 12 (4):2–8.

Hawkley, Louise C., and John T. Cacioppo. 2010. 'Loneliness matters: A theoretical and empirical review of consequences and mechanisms.' *Annals of Behavioral Medicine* 40 (2):218–227.

Henriksen, Mads Gram, Andrea Raballo, and Josef Parnas. 2015. 'The pathogenesis of auditory verbal hallucinations in schizophrenia: A clinical–phenomenological account.' *Philosophy, Psychiatry, & Psychology* 22 (3):165–181.

Hofrichter, Richard. 2003. *Health and social justice: A reader on the politics, ideology, and inequity in the distribution of disease*. San Francisco: Jossey-Bass

Hughes, Gordon, and Michael Rowe. 2007. 'Neighbourhood policing and community safety: Researching the instabilities of the local governance of crime, disorder and security in contemporary UK.' *Criminology & Criminal Justice* 7 (4):317–346.

Immordino-Yang, Mary Helen, and Antonio Damasio. 2007. 'We feel, therefore we learn: The relevance of affective and social neuroscience to education.' *Mind, Brain, and Education* 1 (1):3–10.

Isaac, Kathleen S., Jennifer L. Hay, and Erica I. Lubetkin. 2016. 'Incorporating spirituality in primary care.' *Journal of Religion and Health* 55 (3):1065–1077.

Janoff-Bulman, Ronnie. 1985. 'The aftermath of victimization: Rebuilding shattered assumptions.' *Trauma and its Wake* 1:15–35.

Jung, Carl G. 1933. *Modern man in search of a soul*. Translated by W.S. Dell, and Cary F. Baynes. New York: Harcourt Brace Jovanovich.

Juster, Robert-Paul, Bruce S. McEwen, and Sonia J. Lupien. 2010. 'Allostatic load biomarkers of chronic stress and impact on health and cognition.' *Neuroscience & Biobehavioral Reviews* 35 (1):2–16.

Kark, Ronit, and Abraham Carmeli. 2009. 'Alive and creating: The mediating role of vitality and aliveness in the relationship between psychological safety and creative work involvement.' *Journal of Organizational Behavior: The International Journal of Industrial, Occupational and Organizational Psychology and Behavior* 30 (6):785–804.

Kent, Gerry, Helen Howie, Michelle Fletcher, Ruth Newbury-Ecob, and Ken Hosie. 2000. 'The relationship between perceived risk, thought intrusiveness and emotional well-being in women receiving counselling for breast cancer risk in a family history clinic.' *British Journal of Health Psychology* 5 (1):15–26.

Kezelman, Cathy, and Pam Stavropoulos. 2019. *Practice guidelines for treatment of complex Trauma*. Sydney: Blue Knot Foundation

Kilcullen, M.L., A. Swinbourne, and Y. Cadet-James. 2012. 'Mental health and connectedness: Exploring aboriginal and Torres Strait Islander perspectives.' *Journal of Paediatrics and Child Health* 48:62–62.

Kimball, Cynthia, Chris Boyatzis, Kaye Cook, Kathleen Leonard, and Kelly Flanagan. 2013. 'Attachment to God: A qualitative exploration of emerging adults' spiritual relationship with God.' *Journal of Psychology and Theology* 41 (3):175–188.

Kircher, Tilo, and Anthony David. 2003. *The self in neuroscience and psychiatry.* Cambridge: Cambridge University Press.

Kirkengen, Anna Luise, and Eline Thornquist. 2012. 'The lived body as a medical topic: An argument for an ethically informed epistemology.' *Journal of Evaluation in Clinical Practice* 18 (5):1095–1101.

Koopman, C., S.F. Wanat, S. Whitsell, D. Westrup, and R.A. Matano. 2003. 'Relationships of alcohol use, stress, avoidance coping, and other factors with mental health in a highly educated workforce.' *American Journal of Health Promotion* 17 (4):259–268.

Kuo, Frances E., Magdalena Bacaicoa, and William C. Sullivan. 1998. 'Transforming inner-city landscapes trees, d, and preference.' *Environment and Behavior* 30 (1):28–59.

Laurin, Kristin, Karina Schumann, and John G. Holmes. 2014. 'A relationship with God? Connecting with the divine to assuage fears of interpersonal rejection.' *Social Psychological and Personality Science* 5 (7):777–785. doi:10.1177/1948550614531800.

Lavie, Nilli, Diane M. Beck, and Nikos Konstantinou. 2014. 'Blinded by the load: Attention, awareness and the role of perceptual load.' *Philosophical Transactions of the Royal Society B* 369 (1641):1–10.

Leary, Mark R., Eleanor B. Tate, Claire E. Adams, Ashley Batts Allen, and Jessica Hancock. 2007. 'Self-compassion and reactions to unpleasant self-relevant events: The implications of treating oneself kindly.' *Journal of Personality and Social Psychology* 92 (5):887–904.

Lereya, Suzet Tanya, William E. Copeland, E. Jane Costello, and Dieter Wolke. 2015. 'Adult mental health consequences of peer bullying and maltreatment in childhood: Two cohorts in two countries.' *The Lancet Psychiatry* 2 (6):524–531.

Levy, Barry S., and Victor W. Sidel. 2013. *Social injustice and public health.* New Year: Oxford University Press.

Lucchetti, Giancarlo, Rodrigo M. Bassi, and Alessandra L. Granero Lucchetti. 2013. 'Taking spiritual history in clinical practice: A systematic review of instruments.' *Explore* 9 (3):159–170.

Lupien, Sonia J., Bruce S. McEwen, Megan R. Gunnar, and Christine Heim. 2009. 'Effects of stress throughout the lifespan on the brain, behaviour and cognition.' *Nature Reviews Neuroscience* 10 (6):434–445.

MacKenzie, Doris Layton, and Lynne Goodstein. 1985. 'Long-term incarceration impacts and characteristics of long-term offenders: An empirical analysis.' *Criminal Justice and Behavior* 12 (4):395–414.

Marmot, Michael. 2005. 'Social determinants of health inequalities.' *The Lancet* 365 (9464):1099–1104.

Maslow, A.H. 1954. *Motivation and personality third edition.* Edited by R. Frager, J. Fadiman, C. McReynolds, and R. Cox. New York: Harper Collins Publishers.

Matthieu, Monica M., and Andre Ivanoff. 2006. 'Using stress, appraisal, and coping theories in clinical practice: Assessments of coping strategies after disasters.' *Brief treatment and Crisis Intervention* 6 (4):337–348.

Meares, R. 2019. 'The human brain-mind system.' In *Humanising mental health in Australia: A guide to Trauma-informed approaches*, edited by R. Benjamin, J. Haliburn, and S. King, 31–42. London: Routledge Taylor and Francis Group.

Mount, Balfour. 1993. 'Whole person care: Beyond psychosocial and physical needs.' *American Journal of Hospice and Palliative Medicine* 10 (1):28–37.

Nathanson, Donald L. 1994. *Shame and pride: Affect, sex, and the birth of the self.* New York: W.W. Norton & Company.

Neimeyer, Robert A. 2001. *Meaning reconstruction & the experience of loss.* Washington, DC: American Psychological Association.

Neimeyer, Robert A., and John R. Jordan. 2002. *Disenfranchisement as empathic failure: Grief therapy and the co-construction of meaning, Disenfranchised grief.* Champaign, IL: Research Press.

Newcomb, Michael D., and Lisa L. Harlow. 1986. 'Life events and substance use among adolescents: Mediating effects of perceived loss of control and meaninglessness in life.' *Journal of Personality and Social Psychology* 51 (3):564–577. doi:10.1037/0022-3514.51.3.564.

Ogden, P., K. Minton, and C. Pain, eds. 2006. *Trauma and the body. A sensorimotor approach to psychotherapy.* New York: W.W. Norton & Company.

Pajulo, Marjukka, Nina Pyykkönen, Mirjam Kalland, Jari Sinkkonen, Hans Helenius, Raija-Leena Punamäki, and Nancy Suchman. 2012. 'Substance-abusing mothers in residential treatment with their babies: Importance of pre-and postnatal maternal reflective functioning.' *Infant Mental Health Journal* 33 (1):70–81.

Panksepp, Jaak. 1982. 'Toward a general psychobiological theory of emotions.' *Behavioral and Brain Sciences* 5 (03):407–422.

Paris, Roland. 2001. 'Human security: Paradigm shift or hot air?' *International Security* 26 (2):87–102.

Perry, Bruce D., Ronnie A. Pollard, Toi L. Blakley, William L. Baker, and Domenico Vigilante. 1995. 'Childhood trauma, the neurobiology of adaptation, and use dependent development of the brain: How states become traits.' *Infant Mental Health Journal* 16 (4):271–291.

Phillips, Maggie, and Claire Frederick. 1995. *Healing the divided self: Clinical and Ericksonian hypnotherapy for post-traumatic and dissociative conditions.* New York: W.W. Norton & Company.

Pinstrup-Andersen, Per. 2009. 'Food security: Definition and measurement.' *Food Security* 1 (1):5–7.

Porges, Stephen W. 2003. 'Social engagement and attachment.' *Annals of the New York Academy of Sciences* 1008 (1):31–47.

Porges, Stephen W. 2014. *Connectedness as a biological imperative.* Australian Childhood Foundation Conference, Melbourne.

Porter, Matthew, and Nick Haslam. 2005. 'Predisplacement and postdisplacement factors associated with mental health of refugees and internally displaced persons: A meta-analysis.' *Jama* 294 (5):602–612.

Preece, David A., Rodrigo Becerra, Ken Robinson, Justine Dandy, and Alfred Allan. 2018. 'Measuring emotion regulation ability across negative and positive emotions: The Perth Emotion Regulation Competency Inventory (PERCI).' *Personality and Individual Differences* 135:229–241.

Priel, Beatriz, and Golan Shahar. 2000. 'Dependency, self-criticism, social context and distress: Comparing moderating and mediating models.' *Personality and Individual Differences* 28 (3):515–525.

Reeve, J. 2010. 'Interpretive medicine: Supporting generalism in a changing primary care world.' *Occasional Paper Royal College of General Practitioners* 88:1–20.

Robinson, Bryan E. 1998. 'Spouses of workaholics: Clinical implications for psychotherapy.' *Psychotherapy: Theory, Research, Practice, Training* 35 (2):260–268.

Rothbart, Mary K., and M. Rosario Rueda. 2005. 'The development of effortful control.' In *Developing individuality in the human brain: A tribute to Michael I. Posner*, edited by E. Mayr, and S. Keele, 167–188. Washington, DC: American Psychological Association.

Sampson, Harold. 1992. 'The role of "real"; experience in psychopathology and treatment.' *Psychoanalytic Dialogues* 2 (4):509–528.

Sayin, Eda, Aradhna Krishna, Caroline Ardelet, Gwenaëlle Briand Decré, and Alain Goudey. 2015. '"Sound and safe": The effect of ambient sound on the perceived safety of public spaces.' *International Journal of Research in Marketing* 32 (4):343–353.

Sbarra, David A., and Cindy Hazan. 2008. 'Coregulation, dysregulation, self-regulation: An integrative analysis and empirical agenda for understanding adult attachment, separation, loss, and recovery.' *Personality and Social Psychology Review* 12 (2):141–167.

Scaer, Robert. 2014. *The body bears the burden: Trauma, dissociation, and disease.* New York: Routledge Taylor and Francis Group.

Schacter, Daniel L., Jeffrey Bowers, and Jill Booker. 1989. 'Intention, awareness, and implicit memory: The retrieval intentionality criterion.' In *Implicit memory: Theoretical issues*, edited by S. Lewandowsky, J.C. Dunn, and K. Kirsner. Hillsdale, NY: Lawrence Erlbaum Associates, Inc.

Schore, A.N. 2001. 'Effects of a secure attachment relationship on right brain development, affect regulation, and infant mental health.' *Infant Mental Health Journal* 22 (1–2):7–66.

Shahar, Ben, Erica R. Carlin, David E. Engle, Jayanta Hegde, Ohad Szepsenwol, and Hal Arkowitz. 2012. 'A pilot investigation of emotion-focused two-chair dialogue intervention for self-criticism.' *Clinical Psychology & Psychotherapy* 19 (6):496–507.

Siegel, D.J. 2001. 'Toward an interpersonal neurobiology of the developing mind: Attachment relationships, "mindsight", and neural integration.' *Infant Mental Health Journal* 22 (1–2):67–94.

Siegel, D.J., ed. 2010. *Mindsight.* Oxford: One World.

Slavich, George M., Baldwin M. Way, Naomi I. Eisenberger, and Shelley E. Taylor. 2010. 'Neural sensitivity to social rejection is associated with inflammatory responses to social stress.' *Proceedings of the National Academy of Sciences* 107 (33):14817–14822.

Sperry, Len. 2002. *Transforming self and community: Revisioning pastoral counseling and spiritual direction.* Collegeville: Liturgical Press.

Stamenov, Maxim. 2003. 'Language and self-consciousness: Modes of self-presentation in language structure.' In *The self in neuroscience and psychiatry*, edited by T. Kircher, and A. David, 76–104. Cambridge: Cambridge University Press.

Stolorow, Robert D. 2000. 'From isolated minds to experiential worlds: An intersubjective space odyssey.' *American Journal of Psychotherapy* 54 (2):149–151.

Stone, Louise. 2013. 'Reframing chaos: A qualitative study of GPs managing patients with medically unexplained symptoms.' *Australian Family Physician* 42 (7):1–7.

Sugarman, Alan. 2006. 'Mentalization, insightfulness, and therapeutic action The importance of mental organization.' *International Journal of Psychoanalysis* 87 (4):965–987. doi:10.1516/6DGH-0KJT-PA40-REX9.

Teicher, Martin H., Jacqueline A. Samson, Carl M. Anderson, and Kyoko Ohashi. 2016. 'The effects of childhood maltreatment on brain structure, function and connectivity.' *Nature Reviews Neuroscience* 17 (10):652–666.

Tepper, Bennett J. 2001. 'Health consequences of organizational injustice: Tests of main and interactive effects.' *Organizational Behavior and Human Decision Processes* 86 (2):197–215.

Thompson, Evan, and Dan Zahavi. 2007. 'Philosophical issues: Phenomenology.' In *Cambridge handbook of consciousness studies*, edited by P.D. Zelaso, M. Moscovitch, and E. Thompson, 67–87. New York: Cambridge University Press.

Thurston, Wilfreda E., Amrita Roy, Barbara Clow, David Este, Tess Gordey, Margaret Haworth-Brockman, Liza McCoy, Rachel Rapaport Beck, Christine Saulnier, and Lesley Carruthers. 2013. 'Pathways into and out of homelessness: Domestic violence and housing security for immigrant women.' *Journal of Immigrant & Refugee Studies* 11 (3):278–298.

Todres, L., K. Galvin, and K. Dahlberg. 2007. 'Lifeworld-led healthcare: Revisiting a humanising philosophy that integrates emerging trends.' *Medicine, Health Care and Philosophy* 10 (1):53–63.

Tomasdottir, Margret Olafia, Johann Agust Sigurdsson, Halfdan Petursson, Anna Luise Kirkengen, Steinar Krokstad, Bruce McEwen, Irene Hetlevik, and Linn Getz. 2015. 'Self reported childhood difficulties, adult multimorbidity and allostatic load. A cross-sectional analysis of the Norwegian HUNT study.' *PLOS ONE* 10 (6):e0130591. https://doi.org/10.1371/journal.pone.0130591.

Tuch, Richard Howard. 2007. 'Thinking with, and about, patients too scared to think: Can non-interpretive maneuvers stimulate reflective thought?' *International Journal of Psychoanalysis* 88 (1):91–111. doi:10.1516/D5T4-QMCP-8T4K-0UP8.

Twenge, Jean M., Kathleen R. Catanese, and Roy F. Baumeister. 2003. 'Social exclusion and the deconstructed state: Time perception, meaninglessness, lethargy, lack of emotion, and self-awareness.' *Journal of Personality and Social Psychology* 85 (3):409.

Tziner, Aharon, and Miri Tanami. 2013. 'Examining the links between attachment, perfectionism, and job motivation potential with job engagement and workaholism.' *Journal of Work and Organisational Psychology* 29:65–74. http://dx.doi.org/10.5093/tr2013a10.

Van der Kolk, Bessel A. 2014. *The body keeps the score: Mind, brain, body in the transformation of Trauma*. New York: Viking.

Van der Kolk, Bessel A., and Alexander C. McFarlane. 2012. *Traumatic stress: The effects of overwhelming experience on mind, body, and society*. New York: The Guilford Press.

Vivero, Veronica Navarrete, and Sharon Rae Jenkins. 1999. 'Existential hazards of the multicultural individual: Defining and understanding "cultural homelessness".' *Cultural Diversity and Ethnic Minority Psychology* 5 (1):6–26.

Wallace, Rodrick, and Deborah Wallace. 1997. 'Socioeconomic determinants of health: Community marginalisation and the diffusion of disease and disorder in the United States.' *BMJ: British Medical Journal* 314:1341. https://doi.org/10.1136/bmj.314.7090.1341.

Watkins, Edward R. 2008. 'Constructive and unconstructive repetitive thought.' *Psychological Bulletin* 134 (2):163–206. doi:10.1037/0033-2909.134.2.163.

Wiley, Joshua F., Tara L. Gruenewald, Arun S. Karlamangla, and Teresa E. Seeman. 2016. 'Modeling multisystem physiological dysregulation.' *Psychosomatic Medicine* 78 (3):290–301.

Wood, Stephen J., Nicholas B. Allen, and Christos Pantelis. 2009. *The neuropsychology of mental illness*. New York: Cambridge University Press.

Zhang, Ying, Paul J. Beggs, Hilary Bambrick, Helen L. Berry, Martina K. Linnenluecke, Stefan Trueck, Robyn Alders, Peng Bi, Sinead M. Boylan, and Donna Green. 2018. 'The MJA–lancet countdown on health and climate change: Australian policy inaction threatens lives.' *Medical Journal of Australia* 209 (11):474.

8 *Nouns of disorder* and *verbs of wellbeing*

Noticing dynamics can build Humpty's *sense of safety*

- *Nouns of disorder* can blind us to the *verbs of wellbeing*
- Attending to dynamics and patterns could help practitioners to see growth
- Joining with Humpty to build *sense of safety dynamics* aligns with his meta-need for safety

A key facet of the *sense of safety* framework is awareness of dynamic processes that build, protect and reveal *sense of safety*. As well as maintaining awareness of breadth of the whole person in their relationships and context (*sense of safety domains*), practitioners also need to maintain awareness of dynamics that can build or destroy wellbeing. These dynamics can be visible within the therapeutic relationship, within an organisation, workplace or family system within the person's story. With experience, recognition of these dynamics can be honed, sensitively attuned to, observed as patterns of response and modified or altered. The *sense of safety dynamics* developed through this research and described in Chapter Nine could become therapeutic goals within the practitioner themselves as well as the person they are caring for. These dynamics could also guide organisational goals and structures.

Dynamic processes are much more difficult to describe or measure than static lesions or objective measurements. This difficulty with measuring means they are often inadvertently side-lined or ignored in positivist and technical forms of knowledge. A lack of awareness of dynamics can mean people are related to as objects or machines: whether patients or clinicians, employees or employers, teachers, students, citizens or political leaders. This difficulty with complex dynamics has led to a complicated categorisation of ill health. In some fields it has led to reification: where abstract concepts (such as how the mind works when healthy or what people do when they are fearful) are turned into more concrete representations (such as 'mental health' or 'anxiety'). Dynamic complex processes are therefore simplified and named in a way that presents them as objects, as things, as real entities. Appraisal of dynamics is a relational task – probing, sensing and responding together to discern the dynamic (Gray 2017). This requires trust and honesty. In systems and ways of being that do not value relationships or the time taken to build them, these dynamics are even more difficult to attend to.

At its worst, this process can leave us with a list of *nouns of disorder* (diseases, symptoms, addictions or behaviours) that are seen as 'things' that need to be eradicated or reduced in intensity. Often symptoms and behaviours (nouns) are masked or suppressed using technology – such as medication, cognitive techniques, behaviour management or workplace systems – rather than attending to the processes that contribute to or alleviate these nouns. This can mean sedating someone to sleep might be more important than understanding the flashbacks she faces in her nightmares. It can mean someone's sadness over the loss of their dog who they see as their child can be medicated with 'antidepressants' with little attention to the active process of grief. It can mean that mood-altering drugs can get away with being named for the purported 'disease' they treat, rather than for their dynamic psychoactive properties. It can make it normal to treat children's distractibility with medication rather than face the reality of how disorienting their homes are.

Dynamics can instead be seen as the *verbs of wellbeing*. A focus on the *nouns of disorder* – the observable political and community structures, costs, categories, diagnoses, organs, lesions, microbes, cellular receptors and DNA – has created a particular grammar of the health care system. It has inadvertently silenced the verbs. These verbs include the pushes and pulls of motivation. Both Maslow (1943) and Frankl name the importance of 'motives that pull' (Frankl 1978, 52). The verbs of wellbeing also include expectations, decisions, desires and dreams and the physiological processes of feedback, regulation, inflammation, allostasis and homeostasis. They include the relational processes of co-regulation, dialogue, disagreement, tuning in, and turning towards as well as being available, responsive and soothing. They include the active process of grieving, which Margaret Stroebe and Henk Shut have confirmed as a process of oscillation between 'restoration orientation' and 'loss orientation' (Stroebe and Schut 2010). The attachment literature describes the importance of the delicate dyadic attunement of carer-child and romantic adult relational processes (Schore 2001, Mikulincer and Shaver 2007). Internal family systems, ego-state, hypnotherapy and self-compassion literature clarify the importance to wellbeing of intrapsychic processes of connection and attention. Table 8.1 includes a brainstorm of verbs that may be part of Humpty's wellbeing. When I was writing this list, I read them to my teenage daughter and she added 'to stroll, to fly, to hug'.

As mentioned in Chapter One, the recovery literature, written by those who have recovered from diagnoses of 'mental illness', points clearly to the importance of movement: from passive to active sense of self, from hopelessness to hope, from disconnection to connection (Jacobson and Greenley 2001). Within therapeutic relationships, transference and countertransference are acknowledged dynamics. Relational forms of therapy such as psychodynamic, sensorimotor and couple and family therapies are built on awareness of dynamics. The generalist literature has a dynamic therapeutic goal to increase 'a sense of integrity and wholeness' (Hutchinson 2011, 1), 'enable patients to engage or

Table 8.1 Verbs of Wellbeing – a Brainstorm

to move	to pull	to forgive	to trust	to share
to observe	to push	to comfort	to respond	to activate
to concentrate	to contribute	to soothe	to restore	to care
to attend	to act	to connect	to heal	to collaborate
to notice	to stay	to calm	to reconcile	to nurture
to sense	to leave	to reflect	to forgive	to calm
to discern	to protect	to dialogue	to refuse	to integrate
to organise	to accept	to reveal	to give	to grow
to create	to grieve	to interact	to receive	to engage
to decide	to hope	to offer	to rest	to integrate
to need	to dream	to enquire	to touch	to change
to desire	to perceive	to dwell	to express	to contemplate
to be	to dream	to separate	to make	to create

reengage with their lives as social beings' (Dowrick 2009, 1146). Valuing 'acti-vation' (Hibbard et al. 2004) or facilitating enablement (Howie, Heaney, and Maxwell 2004), patient participation in decision making (Wensing et al. 2002) and sharing power (Stewart 1995) through 'co-creation and co-construction of stories' (Lewis 2014, 196) are all dynamics (verbs) that are therapeutic. The verbs of wellbeing offer an insight into processes that can be excluded from positivist approaches to knowing. They intentionally attend to areas discussed in Chapter Two that can often be excluded from positivist approaches to research and healthcare: subjective inner experience, perception, complex interconnected homeostatic regulatory processes, connected relationship, story, culture, growth and change.

The *sense of safety dynamics* named in this framework are closely linked to stakeholder data and connected and refined by evidence from the literature. As per the principles of transdisciplinary methodology, they remain provisional – open to insights or expansion from other disciplines, new information or others' reanalysis of the data. These dynamics have been named *broad awareness, calm sense-making, respectful connection, capable engagement* and *owning yourself.*

These *sense of safety dynamics* are also situated transcending, connecting and interacting across the seven *whole person domains*. These dynamics are presented in Figure 8.1 below as directions of movement and attention and nur-ture towards self, others and context (symbolised by the arrows) and involving each of the *whole person domains* (symbolised by the concentric circles). They are presented in one image in this figure to remind the practitioner that active processes of seeing, sense-making, respecting, engaging and owning are all con-current parts of the experience of *sense of safety*. None of these dynamics is sufficient in isolation. At times they are subsets of each other, but fundamentally they are all part of an interconnected whole. Each dynamic will be discussed in turn, using data from both stakeholders and the literature (including the new Research Domains Criteria [RDoC] that replace the DSM in US mental health

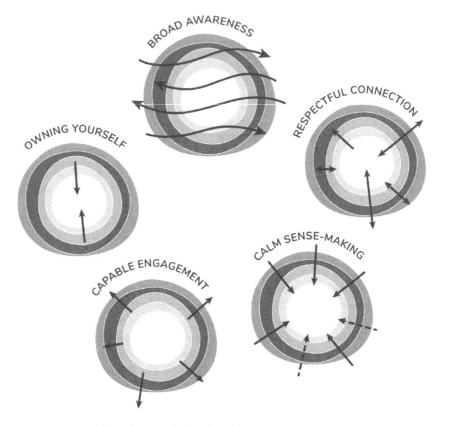

Figure 8.1 Overview of *sense of safety dynamics.*

research) to explain their importance in building, protecting and revealing *sense of safety.*

Sense of safety dynamics are not simply a retreat from risk but a pull towards safety. They are not simply 'being comforted'; they are also about building courage. These dynamics are names for *verbs of wellbeing*. Maslow named an unconscious drive towards safety that involves the whole person (Maslow 1943, 4) and crosses cultures. He said, 'practically everything looks less important than safety and protection' (Maslow 1943, 18). If each practitioner joined Humpty in this endeavour, they may harness innate motivation towards safety as part of healing. Increasing *sense of safety dynamics* is therefore proposed as a holistic transdisciplinary goal of care that might be of more use to people than specialised categorisation and symptom or behaviour reduction. Building a person's *sense of safety* could become an 'overarching purpose' (Kaplan and Maehr 2007, 142) that unifies and directs practitioner approaches to distress. The following chapter will address these *sense of safety dynamics*.

References

Dowrick, Christopher. 2009. 'When diagnosis fails: A commentary on McPherson & Armstrong.' *Social Science & Medicine* 69 (8):1144–1146.

Frankl, Viktor E. 1978. *The unheard cry for meaning: Psychotherapy and humanism.* Sydney: Hodder and Stoughton.

Gray, Ben. 2017. 'The Cynefin framework: Applying an understanding of complexity to medicine.' *Journal of Primary Health Care* 9 (4):258–261.

Hibbard, Judith H., Jean Stockard, Eldon R. Mahoney, and Martin Tusler. 2004. 'Development of the Patient Activation Measure (PAM): Conceptualizing and measuring activation in patients and consumers.' *Health Services Research* 39 (4p1):1005–1026.

Howie, J.G.R., D. Heaney, and M. Maxwell. 2004. 'Quality, core values and the general practice consultation: Issues of definition, measurement and delivery.' *Family Practice* 21 (4):458–468.

Hutchinson, T.A. 2011. *Whole person care: A new paradigm for the 21st century.* New York: Springer.

Jacobson, N., and D. Greenley. 2001. 'What is recovery? A conceptual model and explication.' *Psychiatric Services (Washington, D.C.)* 52 (4):482–485.

Kaplan, Avi, and Martin L. Maehr. 2007. 'The contributions and prospects of goal orientation theory.' *Educational Psychology Review* 19 (2):141–184.

Lewis, Bradley. 2014. 'The four Ps, narrative psychiatry, and the story of George Engel.' *Philosophy, Psychiatry, & Psychology* 21 (3):195–197.

Maslow, Abraham H. 1943. 'A theory of human motivation.' *Psychological Review* 50 (4):370–396.

Mikulincer, Mario, and Phillip R. Shaver. 2007. *Attachment in adulthood: Structure, dynamics, and change.* New York: Guilford Press.

Schore, A.N. 2001. 'Effects of a secure attachment relationship on right brain development, affect regulation, and infant mental health.' *Infant Mental Health Journal* 22 (1–2):7–66.

Stewart, Moira A. 1995. 'Effective physician-patient communication and health outcomes: A review.' *CMAJ: Canadian Medical Association Journal* 152 (9):1423–1433.

Stroebe, Margaret, and Henk Schut. 2010. 'The dual process model of coping with bereavement: A decade on.' *OMEGA-Journal of Death and Dying* 61 (4):273–289.

Wensing, Michel, Glyn Elwyn, Adrian Edwards, Eric Vingerhoets, and Richard Grol. 2002. 'Deconstructing patient centred communication and uncovering shared decision making: An observational study.' *BMC Medical Informatics and Decision Making* 2 (2). https://doi.org/10.1186/1472-6947-2-2.

9 *Sense of safety dynamics* – what processes build, protect and reveal Humpty's *sense of safety*?

- *Sense of safety dynamics* include: *broad awareness*, *calm sense-making*, *respectful connection*, *capable engagement* and *owning yourself*
- These dynamics can build, protect and reveal *sense of safety* in Humpty's life
- Awareness of these dynamics can attune us all to possibilities for healing

The *sense of safety dynamics* impact and interact across all seven of the *whole person domains*. They are active processes (*verbs of wellbeing*) that can be identified across the transdisciplinary literature. These processes are described in many ways, in many disciplinary dialects, so any attempt to describe them here will be necessarily incomplete. They are however patterns that matter. They offer a direction of growth toward wellbeing that can be applied as a wide overarching purpose for facilitating normal development or directing restoration of wellbeing. They are dynamic processes that can build *sense of safety*. Humpty and the practitioners who care for him can build, protect and learn to observe these dynamics in themselves and others.

The dynamics described in this chapter emerged from analysis of stakeholders' responses to the three key questions that have been outlined in Chapter Six and Seven:

What does the phrase 'sense of safety' mean to you?
What threatens people?
How do people sense that they are safe?

This chapter integrates theoretical literature across the disciplines with the dynamics identified in stakeholders' responses and with everyday language that seems to capture the same dynamic. Thematic analysis of interview and focus group data was influenced by Kathy Charmaz's grounded theory focus on verbs and gerunds (a verb which functions as a noun).[1] This focus on observing the action on the ground also aligns with the philosophical orientation of phenomenology. Each of the *sense of safety dynamics* will be discussed in light of stakeholder discussions and the relevant transdisciplinary literature. Each table outlines the everyday language (or verbs of wellbeing); transdisciplinary research areas, including the relevant transdiagnostic phenomena and maladaptive schemata (Wright, Crawford, and Del Castillo 2009) and RDoC domains that are relevant to each dynamic. RDoC domains are presented as an attempt to link the positivist neurological framework of the RDoC to clinical reality, transdisciplinary literature and stakeholder experience (Weine, Langenecker, and Arenliu 2018).

Broad awareness

The *sense of safety dynamic* of *broad awareness* is a form of attention that includes active concurrent intuitive awareness of multiple aspects of self, other and context. As depicted in Figure 9.1 and discussed in Chapter Six, *broad awareness* involves a *broad scope* and *active concurrent* awareness across self, other and context, and across time and place. This awareness is a building block for *integrity* (aware of the self as it interacts with the world), *connection* (aware of self and other), and *coherence* (concurrently aware of self-in-context in a way that protects the whole from fragmentation or inattention). As well as building and protecting, when it is present, *broad awareness* reveals that enough *sense of safety* exists for Humpty to be widely aware (not shut down in survival mode).

Broad awareness is not just awareness of the present or the self. It is fundamentally a sensory process of interconnection and integration. It involves

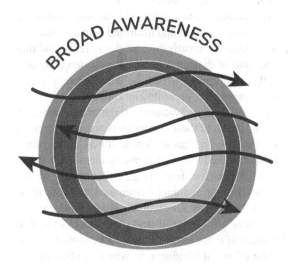

Figure 9.1 Representation of the *broad awareness* dynamic.

interconnection and oscillation between neural networks (Norman et al. 2006), processes of internal and external attention and capacity to integrate prior experience into awareness (Lane 2008, Greenberg 2010, Debner and Jacoby 1994). It requires integrative processes in the brainstem, thalamus, insula and cingulate cortex that contribute to self-awareness and homeostasis (Avery et al. 2014, Simmons et al. 2013). It requires the senses (including interoception and proprioception) (Critchley et al. 2004, 21, Siegel 2010, Glaros 1996, Khalsa and Lapidus 2016) and sensory resonance between people aware of each other through shared attention, intention and emotion (attunement) (Lewis 2005, Gallese, Eagle, and Migone 2007).

Broad awareness is affected by level of consciousness (Damasio 1999), arousal, concentration and 'effortful control' – active directing of attention (Eisenberg, Smith, and Spinrad 2004). It requires internal attention – a capacity for 'constructive internal reflection' (Immordino-Yang, Christodoulou, and Singh 2012, 352) – and internal 'reflective tender attention' (Meares 2000). It also requires the relational skill of reflective function (Benbassat and Priel 2012) or 'mentalising'[2] – awareness of the inner and outer worlds of self and other, as well as the explicit and implicit aspects of communication (Allen 2013, Bateman and Fonagy 2012).

The dynamic of *broad awareness* is described across a number of disciplines. It is part the experience of 'mindfulness', 'metacognition', and 'mindsight' that trains people to increase their 'hub of awareness' (Siegel 2010, 79). It is a healthy 'dual-attention' process – an integration of both right brain (open) and left brain (narrow focused) ways of noticing (McGilchrist 2019, 26). It is part of 'healthy co-consciousness' (Beahrs 1983, 100), a treatment goal for those with traumatic altered awareness (including dissociation).[3] Trauma-informed clinicians call for skills training in awareness: 'patients must learn they are capable of becoming more aware of why they have self-destructive thoughts and behaviours … they are responsible for their behaviour in all states, including dissociative states' (Brand 2001, 138).

Broad awareness is a sensory, relational, neurological and attentional process. It contributes to safety through accurate appraisal and informed decision making, as well as contributing to a sense of humour, creativity, capacity to relate and dialogue, and capacity to hold the tension of dialectics or paradoxes. *Broad awareness* is a fundamental dynamic that underpins each of the other *sense of safety dynamics*. An overview of *broad awareness* is presented in Table 9.1.

Loss of *broad awareness* can be due to scattered, fragmented, blocked, entranced or hyper-focused attention. Each of these processes decrease awareness of the whole – whether physiological (e.g., intoxication or illness); neurological (e.g., dementia or trauma-related altered states of consciousness); functional (e.g., preoccupation or distraction by noise); relational (e.g., disconnection or loss of trust) or intrapsychic (e.g., rumination or avoidant inattention). Derealisation, depersonalisation, flashbacks, amnesia, emotional numbing, dissociation, somatisation, dysmorphic body experiences, distractibility and experiences of self as empty or divided are names for some of these altered states. At its most extreme, loss of *broad awareness* can cause a kind of blindness, a switching off, a forgetting, a numbing, an absence.

Table 9.1 Overview of *Broad Awareness*

Definition	a form of attention that includes active concurrent intuitive awareness of multiple aspects of self, other and context
Ordinary words for *broad awareness*	Having the big picture, on to it, seeing the overview, being present
Ordinary words for loss of *broad awareness*	triggered, lost it, freaked out, spaced out, zoned out, here but not here, numb, flooded, in a trance, amnesia, flashback, distractible, switched off, numb, minimising, ignoring, inattentive, avoidant, unaware, preoccupied
Relevant RDoC domain	Arousal; Sensorimotor systems; Perception and Understanding of Self; Perception and Understanding of Others; Attention; Perception; and Working Memory (Cuthbert and Insel 2013)
Relevant areas of research	Consciousness, arousal, effortful control, attention, concentration, internal reflection, neural networks, insula, cingulate cortex, thalamus, brainstem, mindfulness, mentalisation, reflective function and mindsight (Vanderveren, Bijttebier, and Hermans 2019, Seigel and Hartzell 2003), metacognition, sensation, interoception, proprioception, attunement (Gallese 2006), interoceptive exposure
Research into loss of *broad awareness*	Chronic pain, somatisation, fibromyalgia (McDermid, Rollman, and McCain 1996), trauma, dissociation, pre-mentalisation[4], hypnosis, TRASC (trauma-related altered states of consciousness) (Frewen et al. 2015, Vaitl et al. 2005), maladaptive daydreams (Somer, Somer, and Jopp 2016), experiential avoidance, emotional context insensitivity, alexithymia, self-consciousness, body dysmorphia, amblyopia, obsessions, rumination, flashbacks, cravings, autism
Stakeholder consultation themes	*Broad Scope of Awareness* *Active Concurrent Awareness*

Overwhelming experiences can alter awareness and inner connectedness (Van der Kolk and McFarlane 2012). Those who study the impact of trauma on consciousness – Trauma Related Altered States of Consciousness (TRASC) – note the altered awareness of time, embodiment, arousal, emotion, narrative and experience of other people (Frewen et al. 2015, Vaitl et al. 2005). Studies of maladaptive daydreams[5] note the decoupling of attention from perceptual input creating dissociative absorption (Somer, Somer, and Jopp 2016). *Loss of broad awareness* can impair or distort capacity to attend to one's own feelings – alexithymia. *Loss of broad awareness* impacts unity (and therefore accuracy) of memory, consciousness and identity (Bob 2007). It can also distort attention toward the body – for example somatisation, hypervigilant pain experiences including fibromyalgia (McDermid, Rollman, and McCain 1996), altered self-consciousness (Gallagher and Zahavi 2005) and dysmorphic attention to the body.

Just like Humpty when he sees a snake in the forest (as described in Chapter Five), *broad awareness* is lost in those who have experienced a need to be focussed for the purpose of survival. It can also be lost in conscious or unconscious avoidance of the experience of being aware of frightening or sorrowful aspects of the world, others or the self – 'aversive self-awareness' (Anderson et al. 2018, 3). Restoring *sense of safety* makes *broad awareness* possible: 'the purpose of dissociation is disconnection, escaping reality. Thus, efforts to ground must be accompanied by assurances of safety in the present' (Allen 2013, 87).

A very physical example of loss of *broad awareness* is the impact of the brain not attending to uncomfortable blurred vision in one eye during childhood that can cause lifelong loss of vision in that eye (amblyopia) despite normal neural connections. Similarly, inattention or avoidance of knowing about one's own uncomfortable history can cause amnesia and autobiographical incoherence, which is linked to depressive symptoms, rumination and to loss of reflective function in parenting (Vanderveren, Bijttebier, and Hermans 2019, Seigel and Hartzell 2003). Inattention can also happen in organisations or family systems where only a part of the person or organisation is noticed (e.g., behaviour, performance, words, deliverables) and other aspects of them (e.g., heart intention, motivation, character, morale, culture, purpose, impact on environment) are not noticed. In some highly traumatised family systems, they have not experienced *broad awareness* for generations; for others, it is something they had as children, at times when they felt safe, but they have lost capacity due to physiological, relational and occupational stressors.

As I reflect on situations where I see loss of *broad awareness* in my clinical work, the starkest examples are in those who have been traumatised or overwhelmed physiologically and emotionally. I see this form of disordered sensing when I see a woman who was brought up in a fearful alcoholic home, and yet is preparing to marry a violent alcoholic, seemingly unaware of the risk. I see it in a child who cannot take in the sensory experiences at school, impacting their learning and language development because they remain vigilant, sensing their orderly classroom is as fearful as their chaotic home. I see it in someone whose body has alerted them to pain and who now experiences chronic pain long after the tissue injury has settled. I see it in someone who delays attending the doctor, seemingly unaware of ongoing abdominal pain or other symptoms. I see it in autism impacting capacity to be aware of others in empathic attunement (Gallese 2006). I might also see it in momentary trances during the consultation when someone relives a past experience while telling it or has an intense focus on one aspect of their experience (e.g., pain or self-consciousness about acne) that dominates so they are unable to attend to anything else. I might see it in inaccurate perception within a couple or parent-child interaction where they cannot sense each other's needs, intentions or meaning accurately. I might also see it when someone idealises their partner in a way that is unrealistic (unable to see their dark or unsafe side) and then in another state of mind, can only see their darkness and cannot see the reasons they want to stay connected.

An example from the consulting room of more complete loss of *broad awareness* is a patient who chose to sit in a different chair to usual and presented in a way I didn't recognise with a different tone of voice and posture and none of our usual rapport. When I asked her to change to her usual chair the part of her that I knew better returned with no memory of the last few minutes. Patients also describe these dissociative experiences[6] in their day to day lives. One of my patients packed up her home to move to a new house and found thirty knives she had unknowingly hidden round her home. She had taken a knife to bed to protect herself as a child but did not use it. Ever since, she had determined to be ready to use a knife to protect herself. Each knife represented her unconscious shame at not being able to protect herself. As she realised her decision not to use a knife as a child was a wise decision and not shameful, her dissociative knife-buying stopped.

Loss of *broad awareness* can cause heightened awareness of a negative (or positive) aspect of a person with accompanying inattention to other aspects – losing awareness of their own strengths, resources, emotions, relationships and meaning. Heightened focus on one aspect is manifest in obsessions, cravings, ruminations, flashbacks, somatisation and addictions of all types. It is also evident in hatred and revenge. It can also happen when someone can only see either the injustice and ugliness or the beauty and love in the environment, unable to tolerate being aware of their co-existence. Loss of *broad awareness* might be the key limitation of reductionist positivist science. These narrowed views of the whole are marked by rigidity and loss of capacity to see, acknowledge or adapt to new or alternative information. They impact accuracy and breadth of perception, directly impacting safety.

Practitioners can have functional, relational, neurological and professional reasons for their loss of *broad awareness*. Being tired, hungry, rushed or focused on a reductionist way of seeing or an absorbing or complex task can cause loss of *broad awareness*. They can also be so tuned in to a patient, colleague or child's emotions or beliefs that other alternative perspectives are out of reach. They can become neurologically entranced with feeling sleepy, angry, agitated or hyper focused through countertransference processes that mean they lose awareness of the whole and their own self. Even seemingly straight forward diagnoses like 'depression' can be a hyper focus on one aspect – mood – lose awareness of the whole person. Lack of *broad awareness* limits insights and the potential for options for help and healing for both patient and practitioner. *Broad awareness* protects integrity, facilitates attuned connection and enables coherence across the whole person. *Broad awareness* is something that individuals and groups can recognise and foster in their interactions to order to build and protect *sense of safety*.

Calm sense-making

Calm sense-making is clear headed, intuitive making sense of self, relationships and environment as part of a wider story. As depicted in Figure 9.2, stakeholder consultation revealed it to include 'being aware and clear-headed', able to 'notice broadly, know intuitively' and 'organise and make-sense' of inner, relational and contextual experiences (Lynch 2019). *Broad awareness* (including the themes of being aware and noticing broadly) is a pre-requisite to *calm sense-making*. *Calm sense-making* builds, protects and reveals *sense of safety*. It

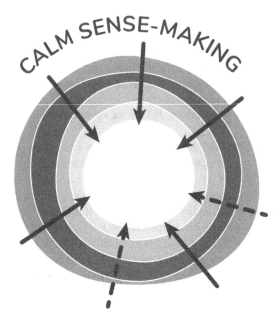

Figure 9.2 Representation of *calm sense-making* dynamic (making sense of self, others and environment).

enables understanding of self (integrity), others (connection) and context. It is a reflective inner process of organisation that is a fundamental building block of coherence. It includes a wide perspective, looking past assumptions or superficial descriptions to be able to reflect, reassess and notice the details at the same time as the big picture. *Calm sense-making* involves physiological regulation (*calm body*), *emotion regulation, co-regulation* in relationships and integrative sense-making (*meaning-making*).

This kind of organising probably starts within the womb as we listen to the voices of our family and hear the rhythm of heart beats. It happens in families through play in our childhood, in listening round the dinner table, in observing and pondering on other's words and lives lived around us. Sense-making happens in music making, in the deep organisation of harmony (or maths), in reasonable argument, writing, reading, image-making and connecting through speaking, listening, reflecting and questioning with others. Sense-making happens when we settle into noticing the rhythms of our breathing (and those we are close to), allow ourselves to align with bodily Circadian rhythms and tune into the cycles of the day, month and seasons of our natural and relational environment. Even rhythms of cleaning, hygiene (Pols 2006), eating and coming home (Nagoski and Nagoski 2020) are ways to organise ourselves. Bodily sense-making includes the way that hormones, immune signals and neurotransmitters communicate through receptors and feedback loops in order to regulate. The body makes sense and organises its response to its environment through homeostasis, allostasis and autonomic tone (particularly vagal tone (Beauchaine 2001, Beauchaine and Thayer 2015, Beauchaine, Gatzke-Kopp, and Mead 2007) (Berntson, Cacioppo, and Quigley 1993)). Calm sense-making happens through storytelling, poetry, metaphor, art, prayer and meditation. Communally, sense-making occurs through rituals and ceremony (Atkinson 2002) (making sense of key life stages and times of day), worship (making sense of priorities), keeping and organising records (in books, libraries, newspapers, history-telling) and creating organisations (ways to order power and responsibility). Morality and tradition based on ancient wisdom literature or on oral traditions (as in Aboriginal 'lore') offer deep communal sense-making over generations. Aboriginal academic Judy Atkinson states 'Lore is clear rules and boundaries. Lore provides a structure for proper behaviour, and creates a *sense of safety*' (Atkinson 2002, 45) (italics added). An overview of calm sense making is presented in Table 9.2.

Perception of threat is inherently disorganising (Scaer 2014, 40). Loss of *calm sense-making* happens when a person perceives threat and their state of mind is narrowed or blinkered by fear. Distorted perceptions (Norton and Hope 2001), alexithymia (Honkalampi et al. 2000), amnesia (Freyd 1994) and emotional dysregulation (Berking and Wupperman 2012) are all forms of disorganisation that both cause and result from fear. Loss of *calm sense-making* can occur through dysregulation of emotion, dysregulation of endocrine or immune processes, loss of capacity to regulate connection in relationships or self-regulate (as in addictive or compulsive coping mechanisms). It can also occur when one's life story has not yet made sense.

I was once consulted by a respected professional who said she had 'anxiety'. At work, she had noticed that she often gave her difficult clients more discounts and extras and later felt dismayed when they did not acknowledge her gifts. As a clinician, my goal was to help her make sense of this. Initially, it seemed random and illogical to her. We sat together, curious about how this story made sense. Suddenly she was surprised by a strong memory of being a six-year-old. As her mother took her and her siblings away from the family home, she decided to leave a jar filled with a posy of flowers she'd collected on the front steps for her alcoholic father. Three weeks later, on a required visit to her father, she noticed the jar of now wilted flowers was sitting on the steps unacknowledged. We spent time noticing her generous heart towards her father and the pain of being unseen. We acknowledged her gift. She started creating glass jars of flowers around her home as a symbol to remind herself that she was seen.

The key elements of *calm sense-making* across the *whole person domains* are outlined below, summarised as *calm body, emotion regulation, co-regulation* and *meaning-making*.

Calm body

There is a beautiful English phrase that has meanings of seeing things clearly, of connecting to ourselves, of becoming saner – 'coming to our senses'. I suspect there are similar phrases in other languages that remind us communally to attend and connect to what we sense as a way to become more reasonable. Implicit in this

Table 9.2 Overview of *Calm Sense-Making* Dynamic

Definition	clear headed, intuitive making sense of self, relationships and environment as part of a wider story
Ordinary words for *calm sense-making*	Coming to our senses, gathering yourself together, or having it in perspective, centred. grounded, insightful, reflective, thoughtful, discerning, responsive, wise
Ordinary words for loss of *calm sense-making*	Confused, disconnected, disorganised, incoherent, reactive, doesn't make sense, fragmented, overwhelmed, discombobulated
Relevant RDoC domain	Arousal and Regulatory Systems (including Circadian Rhythms), and Cognitive Systems (Cuthbert and Insel 2013)
Relevant areas of research	meaning-making, grief, co-regulation, biological rhythms and regulation, allostasis, homeostasis, narrative, mentalisation, reflective function, sensorimotor and mindfulness treatments, modalities focussed on integrating dialectics or increasing focus on underlying values: Dialectic Behaviour Therapy (DBT) (Linehan, Bohus, and Lynch 2007), Acceptance Commitment Therapy (ACT) (Hayes et al. 2006) or Logotherapy (Frankl 2014), Antonovsky's Sense of Coherence Scale, prefrontal cortex function
Research into loss of *calm sense-making*	Multimorbidity, medically unexplained symptoms, somatisation, emotion dysregulation, allostatic overload, distorted perception, alexithymia, amnesia, biomarkers of stress, sleep dysregulation, eating disorders, addictions, suicidality, personality disorders, autoimmune disease, endocrine disorders, deficits in emotion regulation, psychological inflexibility, failure to regulate, intolerance of uncertainty, suppression, compulsivity
Relevant Verbs of Wellbeing	noticing, recognising, reflecting, attuning, attending, discerning, remembering, perceiving, interpreting, integrating, holding, sharing, filtering, mapping and organising of experiences.
Stakeholder consultation themes	Being Aware and Clear-headed Notice Broadly Know Intuitively Organise and Make-Sense
Key elements of *calm sense-making*	*Calm Body* *Emotion Regulation* *Co-Regulate* *Meaning-Making*

phrase is an understanding of the way that senses communicate to us and we make sense of them. Accurate assessment of our senses requires a *calm body*.

Calm sense-making requires calm clear-headedness – a 'quiescent stress system' (Van Praag, de Kloet, and Van Os 2004, 176). The process of calm sense-making cannot happen if the person is in the sympathetic overdrive of 'fight or flight' or parasympathetic overdrive of 'freeze'. There are also bodily processes of *calm sense-making* in homeostasis, allostasis, immune, endocrine and interoceptive feedback loops that are all part of wellbeing. Even pain organises experience, facilitating adaptation to restore homeostasis (Linton 2013).

Normal perception and consciousness are inherently organising (Heller and LaPierre 2012) and are characterised by flexibility, empathy, insight, intuition, bodily regulation, attuned communication, narrative coherence, emotional balance and self-reflection (Siegel 2010, Siegel 2001). Accurate bodily and emotional attunement is a type of 'knowing' that leads to understanding. A fundamental requirement for sense-making is a calm body – a state of mind that might happen around a dining table, digesting, conversing, story-telling, socially tuned in, listening and understanding. A key childhood trauma clinician and neurodevelopmental researcher Bruce Perry says there is a need to *regulate* the body before you *relate*, and only then can you *reason* (Perry 2020).

Emotion regulation

A particularly important aspect of *calm sense-making* is *emotion regulation*. This task of making sense and calming the self is a kind of internal communication, a kind of digesting of experience. It includes learning how to regulate arousal, restore connection with others and understand the personal meaning of experience. This includes being able to name or understand your own reactions and to be able to receive the calm soothing and organising of others, as well as understand and organise the meaning of life experiences. It is part of adapting to and comprehending grief and loss, as well as contentment and joy.

Emotion regulation is initially a physiological process, restoring autonomic homeostasis, to facilitate *broad awareness* and capacity to attend to inner experience at the same time as context. Those who study chronic pain identify the centrality of regulation that is 'in tune' with their environment (Linton 2013). Psychophysiologists note the importance of parasympathetic tone to create an environment for 'social engagement'. This includes facial expressions, neck orientation, body movements and even changing the ear drum tension so that human voice can be heard – no longer on guard for deeper noises (Porges and Lewis 2010). Those who work with the traumatised see emotion as something that can be regulated to be at the right dose – neither too much (aroused and 'off-line') or too little (intellectualising and disengaged). They name the 'window of tolerance' as a goal for each consultation and use emotion regulation techniques such as grounding, distraction and integrative embodied noticing to shift attention and facilitate emotion regulation and sense-making (Briere 2002, Siegel 2010). Emotion regulation is central to wellbeing (Goldin and Gross 2010, Gross 2001, Preece et al. 2018).

Sense-making involves emotion as a form of self-organisation with both conscious and unconscious physiological, social and personal meanings (Rothbart et al. 2011). Greenberg (2010, 1) notes that emotion is 'foundational in the construction of the self and is a key determinant of self-organisation', and Westerman (2007, 324) describes feelings as 'organised action patterns'. This capacity to organise emotions has been linked to learning, attention, memory, decision making and social function (Rothbart and Rueda 2005). Research into the role of the insula and anterior cingulate cortex shows they integrate experience and perception and are a key part of self-regulation and executive function (Ibanez, Gleichgerrcht, and Manes 2010, Posner et al. 2007). Language also has a role in organising emotion (Stein and Trabasso 1992) and in connecting autonomic brainstem and cortical neurological systems. Cozolino (2006, 305), researching narrative and storytelling, confirms that 'narratives provide the brain with a tool for both emotional and neural integration'.

Notably, studies of medically unexplained symptoms and somatisation reveal disorganised responses to emotion (Caretti et al. 2011). Chronic pain is seen as 'failure to regulate' (Linton 2013) in response to context. Threat also dysregulates normally coherent physiological systems – such as sinus arrhythmia (also known as Heart Rate Variability – the responsiveness of heart rate to pressure changes caused by breathing), endocrine stress responses (such as cortisol) and skin conductance. These biomarkers are part of complex feedback loops that link emotional dysregulation to sleep disturbance, psychopathology, eating disorders, borderline personality disorders, substance use and suicidality (Fairholme et al. 2013, Sloan et al. 2017, Beauchaine 2015, Riquino et al. 2018).

Co-regulation

Calm sense-making is also a *relational process*. Social relationships are important to process complex, overwhelming and distressing information (Epstein 2013). As mentioned earlier, stress researchers confirm the buffering role of relationships in shifting stress from toxic to tolerable (Shonkoff et al. 2012). Attachment, psychophysiology, interpersonal neurobiology and mentalisation experts speak of co-regulation (Butler and Randall 2013), 'shared bio-behavioural state' (Geller and Porges 2014, 185) and the 'social synapse' (Cozolino 2006, 6). Relationships can organise emotional experiences (Allen 2013). They confirm the importance of 'another mind capable of resonating, reflecting on, and appropriately responding to the individual's anguish' (Allen 2013, xiii). Although only touched on here, and more fully discussed in the *domain of relationships* in Chapter Seven, *co-regulation* is central to wellbeing and to sense-making in dyads, families, communities and nations.

Meaning-making

Being able to make sense of our world is a uniquely human aspiration (Frankl 1978)[7] – to 'stand back from the world, from ourselves, and from the immediacy of experience' to 'plan, to think flexibly and inventively' (McGilchrist 2019, 21).

Organising experience and making meaning are keys to healing – 'the vitality of the private self depends on the capacity to generate meaning; the inability to generate meaning is a psychic catastrophe' (Modell 2008, 144). *Meaning-making* aligns with Antonovsky's Sense of Coherence scale that sees wellbeing as experiencing life as 'comprehensible, manageable and meaningful' (Eriksson and Lindstrom 2005, 460). Meaning-making creates sense – 'the recovery of meaning in illness and of coherence in one's personal narrative' (Waldfogel 1997, 965).

Meaning-making allows sense – a kind of inner organisation – to emerge from facing the sorrow, anger, fear, hopelessness, connection and joy in your world. Those who research loss, grief and trauma see that digesting and understanding loss leads towards health, while avoiding this process of facing and making sense often leads towards further distress. Sense-making is part of the process of grieving, acknowledging and deeply knowing what has been lost, what is still here and what has changed. Losses are seen as processes that can define who we are as human beings rather than simply being isolated events that are dealt with and then forgotten. Consequently, with each loss, there is both the potential for personal growth and deterioration (Murray 2015). This is a highly individual process of meaning-making – making order out of personal life story (Neimeyer 2001).

Sense-making happens when I listen carefully to myself and discern, amongst a mixture of feelings, what I really think. It happens when I ask myself, 'Is all of me OK with this decision?' Sense-making also includes spiritual and religious approaches to existential distress and meaning in life (Steger 2013, Park 2013, Neimeyer 1997). The human capacity to 'turn tragedy into triumph' (Frankl 1978, 69) gives strength to face existential unease (Tomasdottir et al. 2016), emptiness (Hodges 2002), shattered assumptions about how the world works after trauma (Janoff-Bulman 1985) and even sense of existential abandonment or punishment (Phillips III and Stein 2007, McConnell et al. 2006). Mount (1993, 34), a clinician writing on whole person care, describes the place in healing of 'faith, values, meaning, purpose, inner peace ... transcendent experience of wonder and mystery', and Dowrick (2004, 177) describes the experience of 'eudemonia – well favoured with self and divine' as a way of describing this existential sense-making.

Meaning-making is a creative, integrative human experience (Neimeyer 2001) that is often disrupted by overwhelming experiences, confusion, double binds, paradoxes, shattering of assumptions (Janoff-Bulman 1985) or hopelessness (Lester 2012). Dissociative processes due to trauma cause a loss of internal coherent meaning (Meares 2012) in response to overwhelming threat: 'the organism gives up its unity in order to save itself' (Heller and LaPierre 2012, 147) causing fragmented inner experiences. This loss of unity of self in the face of threat is discussed in more depth in the *domain of sense of self* in Chapter Seven. Loss of sense-making, or a realisation of the 'menacing meanings of their symptoms' (Frank 1986, 345), can lead to depression or the activation of defences, which some see as a natural adaptive withdrawal response to chaos, demoralisation, loss of self-organisation or loss of safety (Blazer 2005, Gilbert 1993, O'keeffe and Ranjith 2007, Cramer 2000). For example loss of sense-making can occur due to loss of culture or 'lore' (Atkinson 2002) as a result of colonisation or migration. It can also occur with disordered morality or moral injury (Jinkerson 2016, Eisenberg 2000), as can occur in combat veterans and other citizens placed in threatening no-win situations. Disorganisation, or loss of *calm sense-making* can be both a result and a cause of loss of *sense of safety*.

Calm sense-making is a key practitioner skill that involves noticing patterns, making sense, *identifying* loss of coherence or order and reflecting with Humpty. These tasks are made more difficult if there is dysregulated emotion in the consultation – 'reactivity and flooding' (Whiting et al. 2012, 30). It is also made more difficult due to the disorder of siloed languages and knowledge cultures of the disciplines. Linn Getz calls us to notice a *gestalt* of experiences of overwhelm (1999), while Jon Allen reminds us that 'diagnosis of multiple disorders potentially undermines a coherent understanding of the individual' (Allen 2013, xiv). Diagnosis of comorbidity and multimorbidity may be a sign of loss of calm sense-making in the health system. Developing a shared understanding of the whole is a key priority of the generalist (Elwyn, Edwards, and Kinnersley 1999, Wensing et al. 2002, Edwards and Elwyn 2009). Awareness of *sense of safety* may naturally engage both clinician and patient in an active process of *calm sense-making*.

Practitioners need skills to manage the 'therapeutic window' (Briere 2002) and make the encounter safe enough so that the person can 'feel without resorting to defences' (Courtois 2004, 421). They can use tools such as the 'art of empathic interrupting' (Fisher 2014) to regulate arousal in storytelling, and they can learn to notice the coherent story that links the whole. This way of seeing assumes an unconscious organisation of the whole that cannot be seen with superficial scanning. As Janina Fisher states: 'the more complicated the client, the simpler I have to be' (Fisher 2014). Trauma researchers note, 'the symptoms tell the story better than the story' (Fisher 2014); 'the body holds the story of what happened and what it wanted to happen' (Fisher 2014). A stakeholder in this research stated: 'Behaviour is language. Symptom is history' (ia). It is the practitioner's task to make sense of this language:

> The symptom picture acts as memorial to the untold story … though wordless, if we listen with our intuition, we can begin to hear the tragedy, despair, and sometimes even the horror of the baby's story in the somatic symptoms.
> (Paulson 2017)

Seeing an order in symptoms also allows practitioners to notice when patterns are disrupted. This is especially important when the person is experiencing internal fragmentation that they are not even aware of themselves – in ambivalence, disordered thinking, delusions, internal critique or sense of self that is divided (Phillips and Frederick 1995). *Calm sense-making* can also help the practitioner to see distress reduction behaviours as reasonable: 'symptom coherence – a client's seemingly irrational, out-of-control presenting symptom is actually a sensible, cogent, orderly expression of the person's existing constructions of self and world, not a "disorder" or pathology' (Toomey and Ecker 2007, 210). Non-suicidal self-injury or alcohol use, for example, serve meaningful purposes including managing overwhelming emotions (Williams and Hasking 2010). The personal and communal environment of each person with its inherent stressors and restrictions, protections and opportunities, incoherencies or fragmented meanings can be made sense of as part of whole person care. *Calm sense-making* facilitates bodily and emotional integrity, connection through co-regulation and coherence through integrative meaning-making. It offers possibilities of creative new treatment approaches that build *sense of safety*.

Respectful connection

Respectful connection is defined as attuned, trusting, connecting relationships with self, others, wider community and country, as depicted in Figure 9.3. Stakeholders mentioned feeling safe in relationships that are *available and trustworthy*, make you feel *tuned in to* and are experienced as *with you/on your side* (Lynch 2019). They noticed these aspects of relationship across the *whole person domains*, including connection to country, community, family, coaches, teachers, workmates, close relationships and connection to self. They also mentioned contextual experiences of respect such as not feeling rushed, being given adequate information and being respected at work.

Stakeholders described the qualities of the person that increased *sense of safety* as *available and trustworthy*: being present, honest, competent, genuine, stable and offering some level of certainty and predictability. *Tuned in to* meant being attended to, listened to and considered valuable ('truly hearing the person's story'

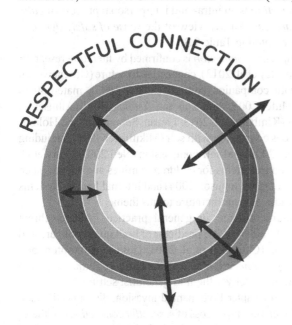

Figure 9.3 Representation of *respectful connection* dynamic (connection between aspects of the self, relationships and environment).

[ia] or 'being listened to and heard with a sense/feeling that they are accepted, and they matter' [mhc]. Having relationships that are *with you/on your side* meant feeling accepted, welcomed and not judged. It included the perception of belonging, trust and meaningful support ('open to listening and open to valuing' [ia]; 'loving supportive attachments in all social spheres' [le]). Although most comments about connection related to being heard and validated by others and being treated respectfully and feeling a sense of belonging and trust, some stakeholders mentioned the quality of self-talk and inner perception of acceptance – being *safe on the inside* (see Chapter Four). The elements of *respectful connection* that build *sense of safety* include relational *coherence* (being tuned in to), *integrity* (having someone on your side) and *connection* (that is available, trustworthy, attuned and offers solidarity).

The dynamic of *respectful connection* clearly defines the quality of connection that builds, protects and reveals *sense of safety*. It also assumes respect for the integrity of the whole – the body, emotions, meaning, culture, identity and environment as well attitudes towards one's own sense of self. This dynamic includes *respectful connection* towards the self as well as interactions that communicate worth and do not objectify, invade, exploit or embarrass others. Stakeholders mentioned loss of internal safety when there is self-loathing and shame in self-talk. They said if 'they don't trust themselves … they've lost that sense of safety within themselves … deep in themselves' (gp). As mentioned in the *sense of self domain*, they used terms such as 'betrayal of self' (mhc) and 'inner berating' (ia) linking it to deliberate self-harm, adding 'it's not safe if you don't like yourself' (gp). In a way, *respectful connection* is an intra- and interpersonal process of *calm sense-making* and *broad awareness*. An overview of the *sense of safety dynamic* of *respectful connection* is presented in Table 9.3.

The broad nature of this *respectful connection* is confirmed by literature researching connection to country (Kingsley et al. 2013), connection to nature (Groenewegen et al. 2006), relationships with companion animals (Siegel 1993), maternofetal attachment (Speckhard and Mufel 2003, Allanson and Astbury 2001, Alhusen et al. 2012) and the transcendent (Kimball et al. 2013, Laurin, Schumann, and Holmes 2014). This breadth also includes connection with self (Mikulincer 1995), including internal dialogue (Lysaker et al. 2003) and self-compassion (Neff 2003, Leary et al. 2007). Current attachment-based treatments for children, families and couples such as Emotion Focussed Couple Therapy (Johnson 2004) and Internal Family Systems (Schwartz and Sweezy 2019) add relevant literature to this theme.

Although personal continuity of care in general practice is under threat (Freeman, Olesen, and Hjortdahl 2003), it is a predictor of both quality of care and patient and clinician satisfaction (Campbell et al. 2001, Guthrie, Brampton, and Wyke 2000). Valuing *respectful connection* as a therapeutic goal may enshrine relational processes and the time to deliver them in generalist settings.

Stakeholders, as mentioned in Chapter Five, named invasion, disconnection and confusion as causes of threat in relationships. Loss of *respectful connection* can therefore occur as a result of invasive processes (e.g., physical violence, internal critique or self-loathing), disconnections (e.g., abandonment, inner ignoring or minimising

Table 9.3 Overview of the *Respectful Connection* Dynamic

Definition	attuned trusting connecting relationships with self, others, wider community and country
Ordinary words for *respectful connection*	Seen, heard, accepted, valued, welcomed, cared for, supported, respected, belonging, trust, predictable, honest, included, loved, self-acceptance
Ordinary words for loss of *respectful connection*	Rejection, loneliness, abandonment, disconnection, ignored, 'ghosted', not listened to, marginalised, excluded, discrimination, racism, invasion, corruption, injustice violence, demanding, manipulative, critical, deceitful, disrespectful, shaming, dishonest, betrayal, unpredictable, incompetent, uncertainty, unknown, unsupported, unheard, unvalued, misunderstood, exploited, self-hatred, self-loathing, deliberate self-harm, suicidal, disharmony, cut off, ostracised, estranged
Relevant RDoC domain	Systems for Social Process – Affiliation, Attachment, Social communication, Perception and understanding of others, Perception and understanding of self (Cuthbert and Insel 2013)
Relevant areas of research	Attachment, co-regulation of stress, infant mental health, Social Engagement System, and neurodevelopmental research, couple therapy, interpersonal neurobiology, Emotion Focused Therapy, self-compassion, connection to country, nature, pets, transcendent, maternofetal attachment, Internal Family Systems, internal dialogue, social inclusion, neuroprotective parenting
Research into loss of *respectful connection*	traumatic impact of neglect and adverse childhood experiences, interpersonal violence, reactive attachment, non-verbal emotional abuse, stress, psychophysiology, objectification (including self-objectification), loneliness, social exclusion, homelessness, subjective alienation, loss and grief, abandonment, mistrust, emotional deprivation, defectiveness/shame, social isolation, enmeshment, entitlement/grandiosity
Stakeholder consultation themes	*Available and trustworthy* *Tuned in to* *With you on your side*

of your own needs or experiences) or confusion (e.g., inconsistent or unreliable connection to self or others – including betrayal and ambivalence and loss of internal unity). These processes can affect sense of trust and belonging towards self and others (Courtois 2004). Those studying suicidality note the key contributors of lack of belongingness and sense of burdensomeness in relationships (Joiner 2005). *Respectful connection* offers belonging and a sense of being welcomed and respected, rather than being a burden. Disrespect in all its forms, including disconnection, ignoring and neglect, as well as invasion, demands or violence, is relevant to this dynamic. Loss of *respectful connection* can include 'connection' that actually dehumanises or invades – such as unrealistic expectations, objectification, enmeshment, silencing or ignoring – what some call 'psychological starvation' (Garbarino and Garbarino 1980).

Further to the discussion of shame in Chapter Five, this dynamic brings attention to the chronic internal loss of *respectful connection* that results from shame (fear of disconnection) that can be embodied as a 'global attack on the self' (Talbot 1996, 13). As was discussed in the *domain of the self*, this has been described variously as a form of self-loathing (Fisher 2014), disowning (Longden, Madill, and Waterman 2012), devaluing (O'Hanlon and Bertolino 1998), disavowal (Najavits, Gallop, and Weiss 2006) or dissociation (Dorahy et al. 2015). The self-compassion literature describes pathogenic forms of loss of connection to the self where aspects of the self are considered 'contaminants' (Gilbert et al. 2004, 47). It also describes inner dialogue that has become 'inner harassment' (Gilbert et al. 2004, 32). Frankl also describes 'emotional alienation ... from one's own emotions' (Frankl 1978, 74). Self–oriented perfectionism (Blatt 1995, Hamachek 1978), body dysmorphic disorder and eating disorders (Ruffolo et al. 2006) can also be seen as a form of self-criticism and scrutiny that is a distorted self-perception and attendant disrespect that has links to psychopathology and suicidality (Gilbert 2015).

There is also loss of *respectful connection* towards the environment and community – 'disconnection from country is becoming a family disease' (ia). Stakeholders described the whole person impact of connection to country: 'connection to country – it's a relationship, it's a body sensation, an experience, and its meaning and spirit. It's a part of defining themselves. It actually is the whole thing and it's different to each person' (gp). Stakeholders also repeatedly mentioned contextual loss of respect such as injustice, racism, 'racism – a constant threat, and injustice, an invisible threat.'(ia), lack of protection, exclusion, corruption and other forms of not having community 'available and trustworthy', 'tuned in' or 'with you, on your side'.

Literature relevant to loss of *respectful connection* is found in diverse fields of research. This includes the violation of objectification and violence (Fredrickson and Roberts 1997), including self-objectification (Tiggemann 2011) and objectification implicit in porn creation and use (Walker et al. 2015, Vandenbosch and van Oosten 2017). It also includes the research into the disrespect and dismissal of 'ghosting' using social media (LeFebvre 2017), the disrespect of personal or institutional betrayal (Freyd, Klest, and Allard 2005, Endreß and Pabst 2013, Otter 2011), loss of epistemic trust and shattered trust (Edmondson 2004, Origgi 2012, Fonagy and Allison 2014, Daukas 2006). Literature that unpacks health impacts of abuse and neglect (Spertus et al. 2003, Min et al. 2007, Grassi-Oliveira and Stein 2008, England-Mason et al. 2018), including adverse childhood experiences (Anda et al. 2006, Felitti et al. 1998, Kirkengen 2010), loss and grief (Freed and Mann 2007, Murray 2015) and subjective alienation (Ross and Mirowsky 2009), is fundamentally relevant to this theme. Research into health impacts of marginalisation and social exclusion (Brown et al. 2012, Wallace and Wallace 1997, Eisenberger and Lieberman 2004, Marmot 2005), racism, discrimination or social inclusion (Carson et al. 2007, Carty et al. 2011, Jackson, Williams, and Torres 2003), loneliness (Hawkley and Cacioppo 2010) and homelessness (Sebastian 1985) contributes to understanding this dynamic.

Reflecting on loss of *respectful connection* clinically, there are the obvious situations such as interpersonal violence and the adverse childhood experiences outlined in Chapter Four. There are also chronic forms of disrespect such as racism, inequity, silencing or ridiculing of personhood and voice in the public square (including online public spaces). Disrespect can be observed and communicated through not attending appointments, running late, being rude to the receptionist, slandering others who cannot defend themselves or cutting off relationships without relational repair. Loss of *respectful connection* also occurs internally (not *safe on the inside*) as evocatively summed up in this patient's description of her inner world: 'I have this life sentence in prison with the worst cell mate in the world – me'.

Practitioners can also observe this dynamic in how people treat their colleagues and other staff and how they treat their children, their pets and themselves. For the family doctor, a key relationship requiring availability, trust, being tuned in and 'with you/on your side' is the parent-child interaction. This is a key place where parents can be encouraged to learn to attune and where *respectful connection* can be restored. Relational safety can be learned – even in those who have little exposure to it growing up – 'earned security' (Saunders et al 2011). Safety can be 'earned' through increased parental mentalising and reflective function (Venta et al. 2015, Saunders et al. 2011) and through training in learning to understand the child's behaviour through tuning in to their underlying mental states and intentions.

Clinicians are very aware of the impact of relationships on physiology, as manifested in the 'white coat' phenomenon where fear of the clinician impacts blood pressure. However, awareness of the quality and connectedness of relationships and their impact on health are often just seen as a nice added extra or 'good bedside manner'. The centrality of relationship quality to healthy development and lifelong wellbeing cannot be understated. Any generalist assessment (whether at work, school or healthcare service) cannot ignore the importance of relationships: are they respectful and are they connecting?

GP stakeholders mentioned creating an environment in the consultation room that was 'able to allow others to safely be who they are and address misunderstandings respectfully' (gp). A person with lived experience described feeling safe if the GP offered a form of connection that means they 'know more about you – not just diagnosis and physical symptoms' (le). In the case of those who are already treated with disrespect in the community, this task is even more important. Practitioners need to be aware of the judgement that those who have been traumatised may receive. Doctors are already aware of the 'heart-sink' patient whose 'apparent helplessness and passivity, her entrapment in the past, her intractable depression and somatic complaints and her smouldering anger often frustrate the people close to her' (Herman 1992, 115). Practitioners need to be aware of their own and others' relational boundaries, carefully attending to language, expectations or attitudes that can communicate disrespectful disconnection or invasion. *Respectful connection* is also a key skill set of self-care for the practitioner.

Respectful connection is therefore a key dynamic of healing relationships and an element of people's life stories that is relevant to wellbeing. Attending to loss of *respectful connection* across the *whole person domains* means noticing the quality of internal connection to self, inner experiences, body and meaning, as well as towards other relationships, community and environment.

Capable engagement

Capable engagement is a dynamic interplay of self, other and context that encourages movement, confident self-expression, engagement and purpose – being *safe enough to grow*. Stakeholders' descriptions, as depicted in Figure 9.4, included a capacity to express the self (*having a say*), to engage actively with the relational, intellectual, and physical environment (*freedom to move, grow and learn*) and a purposeful movement into the future (*positive direction*). The dynamic of *capable engagement* captures the person's sense of competence, movement and expression towards themselves, others and their world. It also includes an awareness of context and relationships that facilitate increased confidence to engage.

Stakeholder consultation (Lynch 2019) adds richness to this understanding. *Having a say* reflects their descriptions of the importance of one's own voice, the capacity to have influence and to express, advocate or negotiate on your own behalf through words, actions or even singing! A GP noted 'a feeling in yourself that you can be yourself and request for your needs to be met' (gp), while a mental health clinician noted 'you feel safe enough to just state your perceptions of things' (mhc). *Freedom to move, grow and learn* included an element of engaging with your own emotions and meaning as part of curiosity, creativity and freedom to take a risk and make mistakes in order to grow and learn. One stakeholder noted that safety occurred when people were 'given the opportunity

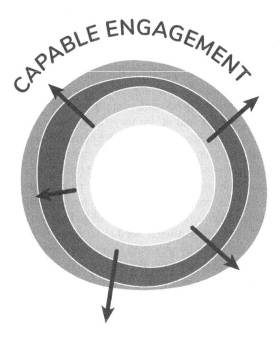

Figure 9.4 Representation of *capable engagement* dynamic (capturing self approaching the world and its relationships.

to learn and "fail" and be encouraged to keep learning' (mhc). It also included a physical experience of movement – exercise, gait and freedom to dance or perform rituals were mentioned – 'being able to move forward and make future plans' (le). *Positive direction* included a sense of movement towards meaningful purpose, a sense of being motivated and empowered to engage or 'move toward' (mhc). It included creativity, pursuing meaning, congruence between actions and values and contribution toward society. Stakeholders included internal experiences of hope, vision, courage and purpose. They included a movement towards meaningful work – 'a positive direction in that it has the most meaning for them' (gp). Stakeholder consultation clearly linked loss of *sense of safety* with loss of movement, the experience of feeling stuck or having one's freedom to express, move and grow constrained by self, others or context. Aging and immobility were also noted to threaten *sense of safety*. Stakeholders also reported a bidirectional experience of inner capacity meeting facilitating relationships with environmental access and opportunity. Stakeholders also mentioned reliable government services, financial back up and management of power dynamics facilitating capacity. Table 9.4 offers an overview of the *capable engagement* dynamic.

Table 9.4 Overview of *Capable Engagement* Dynamic

Definition	a dynamic interplay of self, other and context that encourages movement, confident self-expression, engagement and purpose
Ordinary words for *capable engagement*	Freedom, capacity, curious, growing, learning, engaging, creativity, appropriate risk taking, opportunity, move, dance, sing, advocate, negotiate, influence, confidence, agency, efficacy, able,
Ordinary words for loss of *capable engagement*	Stuck, out of control, insecure, fragile, trapped, constrained, controlled, manipulated, loss of voice, avoid conflict, phobic, ineffective, disabled, passive
Relevant RDoC domain	Positive Valence Systems, including Reward, Effort and Learning (Cuthbert and Insel 2013)
Relevant areas of research	Resilience, positive adaptation, coping skills, post traumatic growth, growth mindset, positive psychology, recovery literature, enablement, assertiveness, workplace psychological security, attachment secure base, self-efficacy, agency, dignity, skills training, outdoor education, approach-oriented coping, social skills training, locus of control
Research into loss of *capable engagement*	Stress, disability, addiction, capability deprivation, hopelessness, learned helplessness, systemic inequity, physical inactivity, autobiographical incoherence, learned helplessness, safety behaviours, experiential avoidance, threat to personal goal, perfectionism, maladaptive coping strategies, injustice, poverty, hopelessness, dependence, unrelenting standards, hypercritical, negativity/pessimism schemas
Stakeholder consultation themes	*Freedom to move, grow and learn* *Having a Say* *Positive Direction*

Capable engagement also has similarity to the concept of 'manageability' that is part of Antonovsky's Sense of Coherence (1993) and the 'Restoration Orientation' of the Dual Process oscillatory model of grief (Stroebe and Schut 2010). Blatz's 'Security Theory' that underpinned early attachment research included an 'experience of adequacy … the individual feels capable of dealing with the situation' (Salter 1940, 6). This also included a sense of capacity to meet the future implications of that decision or situation. Mary Ainsworth wrote that 'Blatz seemed to equate feeling secure with feeling confident or effective, even though one's feeling of efficacy might stem from reliance on something or someone other than oneself' (Ainsworth 2010, 46). This linked to the importance of supportive relationships and what Blatz called 'deputy agents' (Ainsworth 2010, 48) – coping mechanisms that enabled a sense of capacity (discussed further in Chapter Five). Maslow also described this dynamic as a need for 'adequacy and being useful and necessary in the world' (Maslow 1954, 382) and 'confidence in the face of the world' (Maslow 1954, 381).

The dynamic of *capable engagement* is a direction of movement towards others and the world. It also requires feedback from others and the world that confirms your capacity – encouraging environments matter. This dynamic also clearly places *sense of safety* as more than risk-aversion or seeking safe places or people to withdraw to that undermines mastery (Sloan and Telch 2002). Instead, *sense of safety* includes active movement towards more capacity – it includes agency, self-efficacy and approach-oriented coping (Middleton 2016).[8] *Sense of safety* encourages a view of life's struggles as places of growth and reconnection with purpose, recalibrating what matters and engaging with life on its terms. Research into Post Traumatic Growth calls us to 'recognize the power of an adaptive strengths-based model of grief' (Calhoun and Tedeschi 2006, 164). Growth is a 'journey of becoming' (Doroud, Fossey, and Fortune 2018, 118) that involves hope, meaning, discovery, responsibility and participation. Those who research resilience[9] or positive adaptation also describe this dynamic (Walsh 2015, Southwick et al. 2014). The mental health recovery literature, as mentioned in Chapter Eight, identifies this movement or growth from passive to active, from disconnected to connected and from others in control to self in control (Jacobson and Greenley 2001, King, Lloyd, and Meehan 2007). All of these align with the generalist purpose of healing – the primary care priority of enablement (Howie et al. 1998) and 'evidence based hopefulness' (Dowrick 2016) that encourage the 'capacity to act' (Dowrick 2004, 167) and the 'creative capacity' (Reeve 2010, 522) of each person.

Capable engagement can be learnt. As those who research and teach resilience, growth mindsets (Dweck 2010), assertiveness (Lin et al. 2004) and social skills in workplaces, school and families already know, environments can become more able to facilitate resilience. They can become places that offer enough security to encourage creative play and reasoning (Howes and Smith 1995), appropriate risk taking, socialising and enough exposure to challenge to grow. Attachment research also confirms that supportive relational environments predict capacity to step out, explore and discover (Feeney 2004, Feeney and

Thrush 2010). Spousal relationships (Coan et al. 1997, Madhyastha, Hamaker, and Gottman 2011) and work environments that allow self-expression and influence (Edmondson 2004, Ibarra and Andrews 1993) also facilitate *capable engagement*.

Fields of study that address loss of *capable engagement* include those that investigate self-efficacy and agency (Kühn, Brass, and Haggard 2013), physical inactivity (Booth, Roberts, and Laye 2011), passivity in the clinical relationship (Akoul 1998) and experiences of feeling trapped (Milton et al. 2017). Research shows that patterns of trying to cope by avoiding increase revictimisation, auto-biographical incoherence, stress symptoms (Krause et al. 2008, Hermans et al. 2005, Bal et al. 2003) and even back pain (Ayre and Tyson 2001). The self-efficacy and disability literature is also relevant (Woby, Urmston, and Watson 2007, Denison, Åsenlöf, and Lindberg 2004, Lindström 2006). Maslow pointed out that movement and behaviour may not always be towards adaptation and growth; in fact, growth may be shunned (Maslow 1954).

As in the wider community, the clinical environment can take away agency. The hierarchical culture, timelines and even the lack of access to care can cause capability deprivation (Hick and Burchardt 2016) and thus reduce 'basic capability equality' (Sen 1993, 26). The technical fix approach to an objectified biomedical body has replaced the sense of illness as a personal challenge (Reeve, Lloyd-Williams, and Payne 2012). This disempowers the patient, reducing any scope for an experience of *capable engagement* in medical settings.

In clinical practice, as mentioned above, the term 'heart-sink' describes an encounter with someone who has lost their capacity to engage with life. Clinicians understand this term – it reveals the impact of helplessness and hopelessness in family relationships, work or education environments, the wider community systems or belief systems that keep people trapped. Loss of *capable engagement* can be a terrible side effect of chronic avoidant coping mechanisms where each experience avoided seems to confirm the person's lack of capacity to engage.

Decisions made within the consultation can either facilitate or reduce a sense of *capable engagement*. For some people, commencing an antidepressant can be a way to stop feeling uncomfortable feelings that have meanings they don't want to face, or it may mean that they feel flawed in a way that means they feel dependant on the medication for their health long-term. Not every decision is a decision towards growth – practitioners therefore need to be aware of movement towards and away from *capable engagement*. A key element of the dynamic of *capable engagement* in the therapeutic setting is facilitating an environment that is 'dignity enabling' (Gibson et al., 217) where the person can feel safe enough to disagree, to voice their opinion and to take responsibility in collaborative decision-making. In the therapeutic relationship, practitioners also need to be aware of their own and the other person's sense of *capable engagement*. Feeling capable at work is important. Awareness of loss of *capable engagement* facilitated through reflective practice and collegiate discussions is also a key element of safe practice.

Owning yourself

Owning yourself is a dynamic of feeling comfortable, capable and 'with' (aligned to) your whole self. As depicted in Figure 9.5, this dynamic includes physical (*feeling comfortable in yourself*), intrapsychic (*being with yourself*) and relational (having your *capacity acknowledged* by others). It includes personal integrity, inner connection and reflective coherence. These are active embodied and relational experiences. *Feeling comfortable in yourself* was named by stakeholders as an intrapersonal bodily, emotional and interpersonal relational experience, including relationship to environment – being 'able to relax, reduce monitoring my environment' (mhc). The concept of *being with yourself* emerged as stakeholders discussed self-control, capacity to contain themselves and capacity to be grounded and self-reflect with integrity – they spoke of feeling 'safe to be myself' (le). Setting clear boundaries was also be seen as a kind of integrity, knowing what is yours and not yours to feel or do. *Capacity acknowledged* incorporated the sense of acknowledging your own sense of competence, sense of agency and capacity to engage threat and having that capacity acknowledged by others through supportive feedback. It included an element of trust of self, autonomy, control, feeling 'good enough' and 'ok to make mistakes' (gp). The statements 'confidence to be able to cope in adversity' (le), 'agency to address threat … agency to make your world safer' (gp) and 'feeling in control of my life' (mhc) describe this dynamic (Lynch 2019).

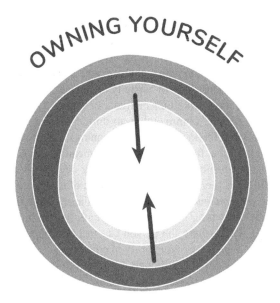

Figure 9.5 Representation of *owning yourself* dynamic (capturing the sense of internal reflective connecting and being with the self).

The dynamic of *owning yourself* includes all the other dynamics – it requires *broad awareness, respectful connection, capable engagement* and *calm sense-making*. It has been named separately in deference to the strong stakeholder endorsement of the concept of ownership (see quotation above) and the inherent risk in medical (and other) settings of losing sight of the patient's ownership of their own decision making and experience. *Owning yourself* is the opposite the of implied societal contract (Blazer 2005) in medical care that allows the patient to relinquish responsibility (Carey and Pilgrim 2010).

The delicate task of being true to yourself and of having integrity while in relationship with other people is fraught with potential experiences of disconnection and the fear of disconnection experienced as shame and loss of self. Learning how to understand and handle your own responses to other people, to have self-control (your own locus of control [Spector et al. 2001]), to maintain your own integrity and remain in relationships is a lifelong journey. It includes being loyal to yourself, growing in comfort within your body and with your humanity and a sense of being able to manage what the world exposes you to. This task is not easy. In fact, Martin Buber says it takes a lifetime to learn how to be yourself when you are near other people (Buber 1923). *Owning yourself* includes this sense of comfort and capacity within yourself.

Owning yourself also includes an attitude of internal relational connection – an inner attitude of 'reflective tender attention' (Meares 2000) or 'inner connection with themselves' (Heller and LaPierre 2012, 202). It involves the quality of inner talk and inner attitudes to self (Neff 2003, Neff, Kirkpatrick, and Rude 2007) and the process of owning your own thoughts (Meares 1986). It also seems to involve a neurobiological awareness that facilitates the capacity to 'integrate a sense of self ... allowing for a continuity of inner experience' (Schore 1994, 33). *Owning yourself* includes movement towards co-awareness, inclusion, welcome and increasing trust of all states of mind (or 'parts' or 'states of consciousness') as belonging to the whole. Working to help the person turn towards themselves, to differentiate themselves from others, to align with their own values (their own true north or inner compass) and to own themselves rather than reject themselves is a central aspect of whole person care and of being *safe on the inside*. *Owning yourself* as outlined in Table 9.5 includes a settled sense of integrity, a capacity for connection and inner coherence about who you are and your life story fits in the world.

Current therapeutic modalities that work with fragmented or disowned parts of self and with self-criticism add relevant literature to this theme. Those who work to increase reflective function of mentalisation (Fonagy, Gergely, and Jurist 2004), mindfulness (Ford 2015), mindsight (Siegel 2010), shame-resilience (Brown 2006), self-efficacy (Bandura and Schunk 1981) and self-compassion (Neff, Kirkpatrick, and Rude 2007) also seem to be working to increase owning of the self. Therapists working with the dialogical self (Hermans and Dimaggio 2004) or ego-state therapy (Forgash and Copeley 2008) move towards a unified owning of all parts of the self. Those who work using the Internal Family Systems model that assumes a need for multiple parts of self to collaborate in owning themselves

Table 9.5 Overview of *Owning Yourself* Dynamic

Definition	a dynamic of feeling comfortable, capable, and 'with' (aligned to) your whole self
Ordinary words for *owning yourself*	Integrity, backing yourself, taking responsibility for yourself, taking on the world, owning up, self-control, self-reflection, agency, boundaried, competence, autonomy, control, strong, differentiated
Ordinary words for loss of *owning yourself*	Disowning, disconnection, feeling stupid, illiterate, overwhelmed by expectations, exposed, vulnerable, powerless, frustration, uncertainty, paranoia, fear of missing out, bullied, victim, shamed, loss of autonomy, psychosis, intoxication, cannot meet own or other's expectations
Relevant RDoC domain	Perception and understanding of self, including 'self-agency' and 'self-knowledge' (Cuthbert and Insel 2013)
Relevant areas of research	patient-centred care, self-efficacy, agency, empowerment, boundaries and self-awareness, reflective function, self-compassion, shame-resilience, dialogical self, ego-state therapy, Internal Family Systems
Research into loss of *owning yourself*	Shame, loss of self-efficacy, victimisation, fragmented self, loss of self-control, bullying, psychosis, vulnerable to harm, failure, insufficient self-control, subjugation, self-sacrifice, emotional inhibition, underdeveloped self schema
Stakeholder consultation themes	*Feeling Comfortable* *Being with Yourself* *Capacity Acknowledged*

would describe this inner integrity as aligning with and being led by your true self (or spiritual centre) (Schwartz and Falconer 2017). Rather than exiled, protective or managerial aspects of self, they note the healing characteristics of self that can lead a person forward. These include creativity, clarity, compassion, curiosity, calmness, and connectedness (Schwartz and Sweezy 2019).

In the context of suffering or illness, injustice or confusion, having a sense that you 'own' yourself is not self-evident, especially if you experience yourself and your story as fragmented (including voice hearing). In the presence of others who disregard your humanity and dignity, including peer pressure, bullying, injustice or violence, it is very difficult to experience your own self as worthy of connection or capable of engaging. Often these experiences physically or relationally entrap people, weighing them down from inside or outside. As mentioned before, internal disowning in the form of the physiologically stressful experience of shame is a form of disowning of the self (Longden, Madill, and Waterman 2012, Dickerson, Gruenewald, and Kemeny 2004). Disowning yourself in relationship to community can be manifested in withdrawal or not taking responsibility for yourself, your actions or your impact on the relational or physical environment.

When reflecting on a clinical story that illustrated *owning yourself*, I remembered a patient who I once kept waiting too long in the waiting room. While she was there, she started thinking about her tasks that afternoon. She was taking her grandkids

Table 9.6 Sense of Safety Dynamics: Definitions and Icons

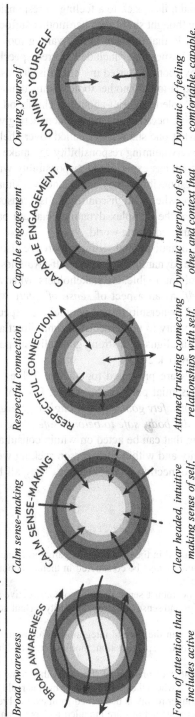

Broad awareness	Calm sense-making	Respectful connection	Capable engagement	Owning yourself
BROAD AWARENESS	CALM SENSE-MAKING	RESPECTFUL CONNECTION	CAPABLE ENGAGEMENT	OWNING YOURSELF
Form of attention that includes active concurrent intuitive awareness of multiple aspects of self, other and context	Clear headed, intuitive making sense of self, relationships and environment as part of a wider story	Attuned trusting connecting relationships with self, others, wider community and country	Dynamic interplay of self, other and context that encourages movement confident self-expression, engagement and purpose	Dynamic of feeling comfortable, capable, and 'with' (aligned) your whole self

to the swimming pool. She suddenly had a flashback to a feeling of responsibility overwhelming her when, as a child, she thought she'd seen her mother suffocating her sister and did not know what to do. In that moment in my waiting room, she suddenly had an altered state of consciousness that included slurred speech and a facial droop. When she came into my room, I started my checklist in case she had a stroke and decided to divert her attention to another topic – immediately her speech and face resolved, and we were able to debrief about her childhood. This is an example of a disconnection occurring because owning and connecting would mean an experience of overwhelm – what one stakeholder called 'overwhelming can't' (ia). Traumatic experiences of overwhelming responsibility can make *owning yourself* very difficult. When someone has experienced responsibility without any authority or capacity to enact that responsibility they are in a no-win situation; they cannot own themselves without overwhelm, so disconnection is a reasonable decision for self-preservation. These are the complex dynamics that are part of learning to own yourself in a complex, unpredictable world.

In the medical consultation or other organisational settings, there are also relational, structural, legal and even cultural dynamics that make self-awareness and taking charge of your own direction feel impossible. GP stakeholders, when asked about the concept of '*owning yourself*' as an aspect of *sense of safety* wholeheartedly agreed, saying they believed ownership turned people's 'perspectives around' (gp). One GP saw it as the capacity to make decisions and direct action and named this as a goal of his care. This aligns with strong generalist support for the importance of the self in health (Dowrick 2017).

These five *sense of safety dynamics* are presented together in Table 9.6 as a reminder they all interact and are essential parts of the whole. Each of these dynamics is involved in the key *sense of safety goals: safe enough to grieve, safe enough to grow, safe on the inside, calm body, safe to belong, safe place to be.* They are all key elements of wellbeing that can be acted on within consultations with practitioners across the community and within each person seeking wellbeing. They all contribute to integrity, connection and coherence. They all build, protect and reveal *sense of safety*.

Notes

1 It is also noted that if something was stated in the data in the negative as a causes of loss of safety (e.g., "injustice"), it would be also be considered in themes about what increased *sense of safety* (e.g., "justice").
2 "Without mentalization there can be no robust sense of self, no constructive social interaction, no mutuality in relationships and sense of personal security" (Daubney and Bateman 2015, 1).
3 Dissociation is defined as "discontinuity in the normal integration of consciousness, memory, identity, emotion, perception, body representation, motor control and behaviour" (Spiegel et al. 2013, 299).
4 Mentalisation theory has named a number of pre-mentalistic states that show a narrowed awareness: "psychic equivalence" (where the person equates mental reality with outer reality), "pretend mode" (where inner reality is decoupled from external reality) and "teleological stance" (where observable actions are attended to more than other ways of knowing).

5 Maladaptive daydreaming is defined as "extensive fantasy activity that replaces human interaction and/or interferes with academic, interpersonal or vocational functioning" (Somer 2002, 199). It can be guilty-dysphoric (associated with neuroticism), poor attentional control (associated with lower levels of conscientiousness), compulsive scene-driven and affect-laden and vivid, causing distressing, time consuming experiences.

6 The DES-II Dissociative Experiences Scale reveals a number of ways this loss of *broad awareness* can manifest.

7 "The truth is that, as the struggle for survival has subsided, the questions has emerged: struggle for what? Ever more people today have the means to live, but no meaning to live for" (Frankl 1978, 21). "If a person has found the meaning sought for he is prepared to suffer, to offer sacrifices, even, if need be to give his life for the sake of it. Contrariwise, if there is no meaning, he is inclined to take his life, and he is prepared to do so even if all his needs, to all appearances, have been satisfied" (Frankl 1978, 20). "Unlike other animals, man is not told by drives and instincts what he must do, and unlike man in former times, he is no longer told by traditions and traditional values what he should do. Now, lacking these directives, he sometimes does not know what he wants to do. The result? Either he does what other people do – which is conformism – or he does what other people want him to do – which is totalitarianism" (Frankl 1978, 25).

8 The concept of "coping" helps to highlight the range of ways that people engage with their world (e.g., act, problem solve, seek support). This framework describes coping as a dynamic adaptive interplay between "stress reactions- immediate and automatic responses to stressful situations" and "action regulation – efforts to mobilise, manage, and direct physiology, emotion, attention, behaviour and cognition in response to stress" (Skinner and Zimmer-Gembeck 2007, 123).

9 The resilience literature also confirms the complex interplay of genetic, epigenetic, developmental, cultural, economic and social influences on the natural adaptive dynamic as part of healthy functioning that is "moving forward and not returning back" (Southwick et al. 2014).

References

Ainsworth, Mary D. Salter. 2010. 'Security and attachment.' *The Secure Child: Timeless Lessons in Parenting and Childhood Education*:43–53.

Akoul, Gregory M. 1998. 'Perpetuating passivity: Reliance and reciprocal determinism in physician-patient interaction.' *Journal of Health Communication* 3 (3):233–259.

Alhusen, Jeanne L., Deborah Gross, Matthew J. Hayat, Anne B. Woods, and Phyllis W. Sharps. 2012. 'The influence of maternal–fetal attachment and health practices on neonatal outcomes in low-income, urban women.' *Research in Nursing & Health* 35 (2):112–120.

Allanson, Susie, and Jill Astbury. 2001. 'Attachment style and broken attachments: Violence, pregnancy, and abortion.' *Australian Journal of Psychology* 53 (3):146–151.

Allen, J.G. 2013. *Restoring mentalizing in attachment relationships: Treating trauma with plain old therapy*. Washington: American Psychiatric Publishing.

Anda, R., V. Felitti, J. Bremner, J. Walker, Ch Whitfield, B. Perry, Sh Dube, and W. Giles. 2006. 'The enduring effects of abuse and related adverse experiences in childhood.' *European Archives of Psychiatry and Clinical Neuroscience* 256 (3):174–186. doi:10.1007/s00406-005-0624-4.

Anderson, Nicholas L., Kathryn E. Smith, Tyler B. Mason, and Janis H. Crowther. 2018. 'Testing an integrative model of affect regulation and avoidance in non-suicidal self-injury and disordered eating.' *Archives of Suicide Research* 22 (2):295–310.

Antonovsky, A. 1993. 'The structure and properties of the sense of coherence scale.' *Social Science & Medicine (1982)* 36 (6):725–733.

Atkinson, J. 2002. *Trauma trails: Recreating songlines. The transgenerational effects of trauma in Indigenous Australia.* Melbourne: Spinifex Press.

Avery, Jason A., Wayne C. Drevets, Scott E. Moseman, Jerzy Bodurka, Joel C. Barcalow, and W. Kyle Simmons. 2014. 'Major depressive disorder is associated with abnormal interoceptive activity and functional connectivity in the insula.' *Biological Psychiatry* 76 (3):258–266.

Ayre, Marianne, and G.A. Tyson. 2001. 'The role of self-efficacy and fear-avoidance beliefs in the prediction of disability.' *Australian Psychologist* 36 (3):250–253.

Bal, Sarah, Paulette Van Oost, Ilse De Bourdeaudhuij, and Geert Crombez. 2003. 'Avoidant coping as a mediator between self-reported sexual abuse and stress-related symptoms in adolescents.' *Child Abuse & Neglect* 27 (8):883–897.

Bandura, Albert, and Dale H. Schunk. 1981. 'Cultivating competence, self-efficacy, and intrinsic interest through proximal self-motivation.' *Journal of Personality and Social Psychology* 41 (3):586–598.

Bateman, Anthony W., and Peter Ed Fonagy. 2012. *Handbook of mentalizing in mental health practice.* Washington, DC: American Psychiatric Pub.

Beahrs, John O. 1983. 'Co-consciousness: A common denominator in hypnosis, multiple personality, and normalcy.' *American Journal of Clinical Hypnosis* 26 (2):100–113.

Beauchaine, Theodore P. 2001. 'Vagal tone, development, and Gray's motivational theory: Toward an integrated model of autonomic nervous system functioning in psychopathology.' *Development and Psychopathology* 13 (2):183–214.

Beauchaine, Theodore P. 2015. 'Respiratory sinus arrhythmia: A transdiagnostic biomarker of emotion dysregulation and psychopathology.' *Current Opinion in Psychology* 3:43–47.

Beauchaine, Theodore P., Lisa Gatzke-Kopp, and Hilary K. Mead. 2007. 'Polyvagal theory and developmental psychopathology: Emotion dysregulation and conduct problems from preschool to adolescence.' *Biological Psychology* 74 (2):174–184.

Beauchaine, Theodore P., and Julian F. Thayer. 2015. 'Heart rate variability as a transdiagnostic biomarker of psychopathology.' *International Journal of Psychophysiology* 98 (2):338–350.

Benbassat, Naomi, and Beatriz Priel. 2012. 'Parenting and adolescent adjustment: The role of parental reflective function.' *Journal of Adolescence* 35 (1):163–174.

Berking, Matthias, and Peggilee Wupperman. 2012. 'Emotion regulation and mental health: Recent findings, current challenges, and future directions.' *Current Opinion in Psychiatry* 25 (2):128–134.

Berntson, Gary G., John T. Cacioppo, and Karen S. Quigley. 1993. 'Cardiac psychophysiology and autonomic space in humans: Empirical perspectives and conceptual implications.' *Psychological Bulletin* 114 (2):296–322.

Blatt, Sidney J. 1995. 'The destructiveness of perfectionism: Implications for the treatment of depression.' *American Psychologist* 50 (12):1003–1020. http://dx.doi.org/10.1037/0003-066X.50.12.1003.

Blazer, Dan German. 2005. *The age of melancholy: 'Major depression' and its social origins.* New York: Routledge.

Bob, Petr. 2007. 'Consciousness and co-consciousness, binding problem and schizophrenia.' *Neuroendocrinology Letters* 28 (6):723–726.

Booth, Frank W., Christian K. Roberts, and Matthew J. Laye. 2011. 'Lack of exercise is a major cause of chronic diseases.' *Comprehensive Physiology* 2 (2):1143–1211.

Brand, Bethany. 2001. 'Establishing safety with patients with dissociative identity disorder.' *Journal of Trauma & Dissociation* 2 (4):133–155.

Briere, John, ed. 2002. *Treating adult survivors of severe childhood.* Edited by J.E.B. Myers, L. Berliner, J. Briere, C.T. Hendrix, C. Jenny and T.A. Reid, *The APSAC handbook on child maltreatment,* 175–203. Thousand Oaks, CA: Sage Publications, Inc.

Brown, Alex, Ushma Scales, Warwick Beever, Bernadette Rickards, Kevin Rowley, and Kerin O'Dea. 2012. 'Exploring the expression of depression and distress in aboriginal men in central Australia: A qualitative study.' *BMC Psychiatry* 12 (97). https://doi.org /10.1186/1471-244X-12-97.

Brown, Brené. 2006. 'Shame resilience theory: A grounded theory study on women and shame.' *Families in Society: The Journal of Contemporary Social Services* 87 (1):43–52.

Buber, Martin. 1923 *I and Thou.* Edinburgh: T & T Clark.

Butler, Emily A., and Ashley K. Randall. 2013. 'Emotional coregulation in close relationships.' *Emotion Review* 5 (2):202–210.

Campbell, S., et al. 2001. 'Identifying predictors of high quality care in English general practice: observational study.' *BMJ* 323 (7316):784.

Calhoun, L.G., and R.G. Tedeschi, eds. 2006. *Handbook of posttraumatic growth. Research and practice.* Mahwah, NJ: Lawrence Erlbaum Associates.

Caretti, Vincenzo, Piero Porcelli, Luigi Solano, Adriano Schimmenti, R. Michael Bagby, and Graeme J. Taylor. 2011. 'Reliability and validity of the Toronto Structured Interview for Alexithymia in a mixed clinical and nonclinical sample from Italy.' *Psychiatry Research* 187 (3):432–436.

Carey, Timothy A., and David Pilgrim. 2010. 'Diagnosis and formulation: What should we tell the students?' *Clinical Psychology & Psychotherapy* 17 (6):447–454.

Carson, Bronwyn, Terry Dunbar, Richard D. Chenhall, and Ross Bailie. 2007. *Social determinants of indigenous health.* Crows Nest: Allen & Unwin.

Carty, Denise C., Daniel J. Kruger, Tonya M. Turner, Bettina Campbell, E. Hill DeLoney, and E. Yvonne Lewis. 2011. 'Racism, health status, and birth outcomes: Results of a participatory community-based intervention and health survey.' *Journal of Urban Health* 88 (1):84–97.

Coan, James, John M Gottman, Julia Babcock, and Neil Jacobson. 1997. 'Battering and the male rejection of influence from women.' *Aggressive Behavior: Official Journal of the International Society for Research on Aggression* 23 (5):375–388.

Courtois, C.A. 2004. 'Complex trauma, complex reactions: Assessment and treatment.' *Psychotherapy: Theory, Research, Practice, Training* 41 (4):412–425.

Cozolino, Louis, ed. 2006. *The neuroscience of human relationships. Attachment and the developing social brain.* New York: W.W. Norton and Company.

Cramer, Phebe. 2000. 'Defense mechanisms in psychology today: Further processes for adaptation.' *American Psychologist* 55 (6):637–646.

Critchley, Hugo D., Stefan Wiens, Pia Rotshtein, Arne Öhman, and Raymond J. Dolan. 2004. 'Neural systems supporting interoceptive awareness.' *Nature Neuroscience* 7 (2):189–195.

Cuthbert, Bruce N., and Thomas R. Insel. 2013. Toward the future of psychiatric diagnosis: The seven pillars of RDoC. *BMC Medicine* 11 (126). Accessed 15/10/16. https://doi.org /10.1186/1741-7015-11-126.

Damasio, Antonio R. 1999. *The feeling of what happens: Body and emotion in the making of consciousness.* New York: Houghton Mifflin Harcourt.

Daubney, Michael, and Anthony Bateman. 2015. 'Mentalization-based therapy (MBT): An overview.' *Australasian Psychiatry* 23 (2):132–135.

Daukas, Nancy. 2006. 'Epistemic trust and social location.' *Episteme* 3 (1–2):109–124.

Debner, James A., and Larry L. Jacoby. 1994. 'Unconscious perception: Attention, awareness, and control.' *Journal of Experimental Psychology: Learning, Memory, and Cognition* 20 (2):304–317.

Denison, Eva, P. Åsenlöf, and P. Lindberg. 2004. 'Self-efficacy, fear avoidance, and pain intensity as predictors of disability in subacute and chronic musculoskeletal pain patients in primary health care.' *Pain* 111 (3):245–252.

Dickerson, Sally S., Tara L. Gruenewald, and Margaret E. Kemeny. 2004. 'When the social self is threatened: Shame, physiology, and health.' *Journal of Personality* 72 (6):1191–1216.

Dorahy, Martin J., Warwick Middleton, Lenaire Seager, Patrick McGurrin, Mary Williams, and Ron Chambers. 2015. 'Dissociation, shame, complex PTSD, child maltreatment and intimate relationship self-concept in dissociative disorder, chronic PTSD and mixed psychiatric groups.' *Journal of Affective Disorders* 172:195–203.

Doroud, Nastaran, Ellie Fossey, and Tracy Fortune. 2018. 'Place for being, doing, becoming and belonging: A meta-synthesis exploring the role of place in mental health recovery.' *Health & Place* 52:110–120.

Dowrick, Christopher. 2004. *Beyond depression: A new approach to understanding and management.* London: Oxford University Press.

Dowrick, Christopher. 2016. 'Suffering and hope: Third Helen Lester memorial lecture.' *Society of Academic Primary Care, Dublin Castle*, 6 July.

Dowrick, Christopher. 2017. *Person-centred primary care: Searching for the self.* London: Routledge.

Dweck, Carol S. 2010. 'Even geniuses work hard.' *Educational Leadership* 68 (1):16–20.

Edmondson, Amy. 2004. 'Psychological safety, trust and learning in organisation: A group-level lens.' In *Trust and distrust in organisations: Dilemmas and approaches*, edited by R.M. Kramer, and K.S. Cook, 239–272. New York: Russell Sage Foundation.

Edwards, Adrian, and Glyn Elwyn. 2009. *Shared decision-making in health care: Achieving evidence-based patient choice.* Oxford: Oxford University Press.

Eisenberg, Nancy. 2000. 'Emotion, regulation, and moral development.' *Annual Review of Psychology* 51 (1):665–697.

Eisenberg, Nancy, Cynthia L. Smith, and Tracy L. Spinrad. 2004. 'Effortful control: Relations with emotion regulation, adjustment, and socialization in childhood.' In *Handbook of self-regulation: Research, theory, and applications*, edited by Roy F. Baumeister, and D. Kathleen Vohs, 259–283. New York: The Guildford Press.

Eisenberger, Naomi I., and Matthew D. Lieberman. 2004. 'Why rejection hurts: A common neural alarm system for physical and social pain.' *Trends in Cognitive Sciences* 8 (7):294–300.

Elwyn, Glyn, Adrian Edwards, and Paul Kinnersley. 1999. 'Shared decision-making in primary care: The neglected second half of the consultation.' *British Journal of General Practice* 49 (443):477–482.

Endreß, Martin, and Andrea Pabst. 2013. 'Violence and shattered trust: Sociological considerations.' *Human Studies* 36 (1):89–106.

England-Mason, Gillian, Rebecca Casey, Mark Ferro, Harriet L. MacMillan, Lil Tonmyr, and Andrea Gonzalez. 2018. 'Child maltreatment and adult multimorbidity: Results from the Canadian Community Health Survey.' *Canadian Journal of Public Health* 109:561–572. https://doi.org/10.17269/s41997-018-0069-y.

Epstein, Ronald Mark. 2013. 'Whole mind and shared mind in clinical decision-making.' *Patient Education and Counseling* 90 (2):200–206.

Eriksson, M., and B. Lindstrom. 2005. 'Validity of Antonovsky's sense of coherence scale: A systematic review.' *Journal of Epidemiology and Community Health* 59 (6):460–466. doi:10.1136/jech.2003.018085.

Fairholme, Christopher P., Elizabeth L. Nosen, Yael I. Nillni, Julie A. Schumacher, Matthew T. Tull, and Scott F. Coffey. 2013. 'Sleep disturbance and emotion dysregulation as transdiagnostic processes in a comorbid sample.' *Behaviour Research and Therapy* 51 (9):540–546.

Feeney, Brooke C. 2004. 'A secure base: Responsive support of goal strivings and exploration in adult intimate relationships.' *Journal of Personality and Social Psychology* 87 (5):631–648. doi:10.1037/0022-3514.87.5.631.

Feeney, Brooke C., and Roxanne L. Thrush. 2010. 'Relationship influences on exploration in adulthood: The characteristics and function of a secure base.' *Journal of Personality and Social Psychology* 98 (1):57–76. doi:10.1037/a0016961.

Felitti, V.J., R.F. Anda, D. Nordenberg, D.F. Williamson, A.M. Spitz, V. Edwards, M.P. Koss, and J.S. Marks. 1998. 'Relationship of childhood abuse and household dysfunction to many of the leading causes of death in adults: The Adverse Childhood Experiences (ACE) study.' *American Journal of Preventive Medicine* 14 (4):245–258.

Fisher, J. 2014. *Transforming Trauma-related shame and self loathing*. Overcoming trauma-related shame and self-loathing Conference, Brisbane.

Fonagy, Peter, and Elizabeth Allison. 2014. 'The role of mentalizing and epistemic trust in the therapeutic relationship.' *Psychotherapy* 51 (3):372–380. doi: 10.1037/a0036505.

Fonagy, Peter, Gyorgy Gergely, and Elliot L. Jurist. 2004. *Affect regulation, mentalization and the development of the self*. New York: Karnac Books.

Ford, Elizabeth E. 2015. *A test of self-compassion as a mediator of the beneficial effects of mindfulness on wellbeing*. Honours Thesis, School of Psychology, The University of Queensland, School of Psychology.

Forgash, Carol Ed, and Margaret Ed Copeley. 2008. *Healing the heart of trauma and dissociation with EMDR and ego state therapy*. New York: Springer Publishing Co.

Frank, J.D. 1986. 'Psychotherapy--the transformation of meanings: Discussion paper.' *Journal of the Royal Society of Medicine* 79 (6):341–346.

Frankl, Viktor E. 1978. *The unheard cry for meaning: Psychotherapy and humanism*. Sydney: Hodder and Stoughton.

Frankl, Viktor E. 2014. *The will to meaning: Foundations and applications of logotherapy*. New York: Penguin.

Fredrickson, Barbara L., and Tomi-Ann Roberts. 1997. 'Objectification theory: Toward understanding women's lived experiences and mental health risks.' *Psychology of Women Quarterly* 21 (2):173–206.

Freed, P.J., and J.J. Mann. 2007. 'Sadness and loss: Toward a neurobiopsychosocial model.' *American Journal of Psychiatry* 164 (1):28–34.

Freeman, G.K., F. Olesen, and P. Hjortdahl. 2003. 'Continuity of care: an essential element of modern general practice?' *Family Practice* 20 (6):623–627.

Frewen, Paul, Kathy Hegadoren, Nick J. Coupland, Brian H. Rowe, Richard W.J. Neufeld, and Ruth Lanius. 2015. 'Trauma related altered states of consciousness (TRASC) and functional impairment 1: Prospective study in acutely traumatized persons.' *Journal of Trauma & Dissociation* 16 (5):500–519. doi:10.1080/15299732.2015.1022925.

Freyd, Jennifer J. 1994. 'Betrayal trauma: Traumatic amnesia as an adaptive response to childhood abuse.' *Ethics & Behavior* 4 (4):307–329.

Freyd, Jennifer J., B. Klest, and C.B. Allard. 2005. 'Betrayal trauma: Relationship to physical health, psychological distress, and a written disclosure intervention.' *Journal of Trauma & Dissociation* 6 (3):83–104.

Gallagher, Shaun, and Dan Zahavi. 2005. 'Phenomenological approaches to self-consciousness.' In *Stanford encyclopaedia of philosophy*, edited by E.N. Zalta. Stanford University: Metaphysics Research Lab. https://plato.stanford.edu/entries/self-consciousness-phenomenological/ https://plato.stanford.edu/cite.html

Gallese, Vittorio. 2006. 'Intentional attunement: A neurophysiological perspective on social cognition and its disruption in autism.' *Brain Research* 1079 (1):15–24.

Gallese, Vittorio, Morris N. Eagle, and Paolo Migone. 2007. 'Intentional attunement: Mirror neurons and the neural underpinnings of interpersonal relations.' *Journal of the American Psychoanalytic Association* 55 (1):131–175.

Garbarino, James, and Anne C. Garbarino. 1980. Emotional maltreatment of children. National Committee for Prevention of Child Abuse.

Geller, Shari M., and Stephen W. Porges. 2014. 'Therapeutic presence: Neurophysiological mechanisms mediating feeling safe in therapeutic relationships.' *Journal of Psychotherapy Integration* 24 (3):178–192.

Getz, Linn. 1999. '"Unexplainable" medical histories and childhood sexual abuse: New doctoral thesis tells you how to investigate the links.' *Scandinavian Journal of Primary Health Care* 17 (2):68–71.

Gibson, Barbara E., Barbara Secker, Debbie Rolfe, Frank Wagner, Bob Parke, and Bhavnita Mistry. 2012. 'Disability and dignity-enabling home environments.' *Social Science & Medicine* 74 (2):211–219.

Gilbert, Paul. 1993. 'Defence and safety: Their function in social behaviour and psychopathology.' *British Journal of Clinical Psychology* 32 (2):131–153.

Gilbert, Paul. 2015. 'Self-disgust, self-hatred, and compassion-focused therapy.' Philip A. Powell, Paul G. Overton, and Jane Simpson. In *The revolting self: Perspectives on the psychological, social, and clinical implications of self-directed disgust*, edited by Philip A. Powell, Paul G. Overton, and Jane Simpson, 223–242. London: Karnac Books Ltd.

Gilbert, Paul, M. Clarke, Susanne Hempel, Jeremy N.V. Miles, and Chris Irons. 2004. 'Criticizing and reassuring oneself: An exploration of forms, styles and reasons in female students.' *British Journal of Clinical Psychology* 43 (1):31–50.

Glaros, Alan G. 1996. 'Awareness of physiological responding under stress and nonstress conditions in temporomandibular disorders.' *Biofeedback and Self-Regulation* 21 (3):261–272.

Goldin, Philippe R., and James J. Gross. 2010. 'Effects of mindfulness-based stress reduction (MBSR) on emotion regulation in social anxiety disorder.' *Emotion* 10 (1):83–91.

Grassi-Oliveira, Rodrigo, and Lilian Milnitsky Stein. 2008. 'Childhood maltreatment associated with PTSD and emotional distress in low-income adults: The burden of neglect.' *Child Abuse & Neglect* 32 (12):1089–1094.

Greenberg, Leslie S. 2010. 'Emotion-focused therapy: A clinical synthesis.' *Focus* 8 (1):32–42.

Groenewegen, Peter P., Agnes E. Van den Berg, Sjerp De Vries, and Robert A. Verheij. 2006. 'Vitamin G: Effects of green space on health, well-being, and social safety.' *BMC Public Health* 6 (149). https://doi.org/10.1186/1471-2458-6-149.

Gross, James J. 2001. 'Emotion regulation in adulthood: Timing is everything.' *Current Directions in Psychological Science* 10 (6):214–219.

Guthrie, B., S. Brampton, and S. Wyke. 2000. 'Does continuity in general practice really matter? Commentary: A patient's perspective of continuity.' *BMJ* 321 (7263):734–736.

Hamachek, Don E. 1978. 'Psychodynamics of normal and neurotic perfectionism.' *Psychology: A Journal of Human Behavior* 15 (1):27–33.

Hawkley, Louise C., and John T. Cacioppo. 2010. 'Loneliness matters: A theoretical and empirical review of consequences and mechanisms.' *Annals of Behavioral Medicine* 40 (2):218–227.

Hayes, Steven C., Jason B. Luoma, Frank W. Bond, Akihiko Masuda, and Jason Lillis. 2006. 'Acceptance and commitment therapy: Model, processes and outcomes.' *Behaviour Research and Therapy* 44 (1):1–25.

Heller, Laurence, and A. LaPierre. 2012. *Healing developmental trauma: How Early Trauma affects self-regulation, self-image, and the capacity for relationship*. Berkeley: North Atlantic Books.

Herman, Judith L. 1992. *Trauma and recovery: From domestic abuse to political terror*. London: Pandora HarpersCollins Publishers Inc.

Hermans, Dirk, Annemie Defranc, Filip Raes, J. Mark G. Williams, and Paul Eelen. 2005. 'Reduced autobiographical memory specificity as an avoidant coping style.' *British Journal of Clinical Psychology* 44 (4):583–589.

Hermans, Hubert J.M., and Giancarlo Dimaggio. 2004. *The dialogical self in psychotherapy: An introduction*. Hove: Brunner Routledge.

Hick, Rod, and Tania Burchardt. 2016. 'Capability deprivation.' In *The Oxford handbook of the social science of poverty*, edited by D. Brady, and L.M. Burton. Vol 75. Oxford Handbooks Online.

Hodges, Shannon. 2002. 'Mental health, depression, and dimensions of spirituality and religion.' *Journal of Adult Development* 9 (2):109–115.

Honkalampi, Kirsi, Jukka Hintikka, Antti Tanskanen, Johannes Lehtonen, and Heimo Viinamäki. 2000. 'Depression is strongly associated with alexithymia in the general population.' *Journal of Psychosomatic Research* 48 (1):99–104.

Howes, Carollee, and Ellen W. Smith. 1995. 'Relations among child care quality, teacher behavior, children's play activities, emotional security, and cognitive activity in child care.' *Early Childhood Research Quarterly* 10 (4):381–404.

Howie, J.G., David J. Heaney, Margaret Maxwell, and Jeremy J. Walker. 1998. 'A comparison of a patient enablement instrument (PEI) against two established satisfaction scales as an outcome measure of primary care consultations.' *Family Practice* 15 (2):165–171.

Ibanez, Agustin, Ezequiel Gleichgerrcht, and Facundo Manes. 2010. 'Clinical effects of insular damage in humans.' *Brain Structure and Function* 214 (5–6):397–410.

Ibarra, Herminia, and Steven B. Andrews. 1993. 'Power, social influence, and sense making: Effects of network centrality and proximity on employee perceptions.' *Administrative Science Quarterly* 38 (2):277–303.

Immordino-Yang, Mary Helen, Joanna A. Christodoulou, and Vanessa Singh. 2012. 'Rest is not idleness implications of the brain's default mode for human development and education.' *Perspectives on Psychological Science* 7 (4):352–364.

Jackson, James S., David R. Williams, and Myriam Torres. 2003. 'Perceptions of discrimination, health and mental health: The social stress process.' In *Social stressors, personal and social resources, and their mental health consequences*, edited by A. Rockville and M.D. Maney, 86–146. Bethesda MD: National Institute of Mental Health.

Jacobson, N., and D. Greenley. 2001. 'What is recovery? A conceptual model and explication.' *Psychiatric Services (Washington, D.C.)* 52 (4):482–485.

Janoff-Bulman, Ronnie. 1985. 'The aftermath of victimization: Rebuilding shattered assumptions.' *Trauma and its Wake* 1:15–35.

Jinkerson, Jeremy D. 2016. 'Defining and assessing moral injury: A syndrome perspective.' *Traumatology* 22 (2):122–130.

Johnson, Sue. 2004. 'An antidote to posttraumatic stress disorder: The creation of secure attachment in couples therapy.' In *Attachment issues in psychopathology and intervention*, edited by L. Atkinson and S. Goldberg, 207–228. London: Lawrence Erbaum Associates.

Joiner, Thomas. 2005. *Why people die by suicide*. London: Harvard University Press.

Khalsa, Sahib S., and Rachel C. Lapidus. 2016. 'Can interoception improve the pragmatic search for biomarkers in psychiatry?' *Frontiers in Psychiatry* 7 (121):1–19. https://doi.org/10.3389/fpsyt.2016.00121.

Kimball, Cynthia, Chris Boyatzis, Kaye Cook, Kathleen Leonard, and Kelly Flanagan. 2013. 'Attachment to God: A qualitative exploration of emerging adults' spiritual relationship with God.' *Journal of Psychology and Theology* 41 (3):175–188.

King, Robert, Chris Lloyd, and Tom Meehan, eds. 2007. *Handbook of psychosocial rehabilitation*. Melbourne: Blackwell Publishing.

Kingsley, Jonathan, Mardie Townsend, Claire Henderson-Wilson, and Bruce Bolam. 2013. 'Developing an exploratory framework linking Australian aboriginal peoples' connection to country and concepts of wellbeing.' *International Journal of Environmental Research and Public Health* 10 (2):678–698.

Kirkengen, Anna Luise. 2010. *The lived experience of violation: How abused children become unhealthy adults*. Vol. 1. Bucharest: Zeta Books.

Krause, Elizabeth D., Stacey Kaltman, Lisa A. Goodman, and Mary Ann Dutton. 2008. 'Avoidant coping and PTSD symptoms related to domestic violence exposure: A longitudinal study.' *Journal of Traumatic Stress* 21 (1):83–90.

Kühn, Simone, Marcel Brass, and Patrick Haggard. 2013. 'Feeling in control: Neural correlates of experience of agency.' *Cortex* 49 (7):1935–1942.

Lane, Richard D. 2008. 'Neural substrates of implicit and explicit emotional processes: A unifying framework for psychosomatic medicine.' *Psychosomatic Medicine* 70 (2):214–231.

Laurin, Kristin, Karina Schumann, and John G. Holmes. 2014. 'A relationship with God? Connecting with the divine to assuage fears of interpersonal rejection.' *Social Psychological and Personality Science* 5 (7):777–785. doi:10.1177/1948550614531800.

Leary, Mark R., Eleanor B. Tate, Claire E. Adams, Ashley Batts Allen, and Jessica Hancock. 2007. 'Self-compassion and reactions to unpleasant self-relevant events: The implications of treating oneself kindly.' *Journal of Personality and Social Psychology* 92 (5):887–904.

LeFebvre, L. 2017. 'Ghosting as a relationship dissolution strategy in the technological age.' In *The impact of social media in modern romantic relationships*, edited by N.M. Punyanunt-Carter, and J.S. Wrench, 219–235. New York: Lexington Books.

Lester, David. 2012. 'Defeat and entrapment as predictors of depression and suicidal ideation versus hopelessness and helplessness.' *Psychological Reports* 111 (2):498–501.

Lewis, Marc D. 2005. 'Getting emotional: A neural perspective on emotion, intention, and consciousness.' *Journal of Consciousness Studies* 12 (8–9):210–235.

Lin, Yen-Ru, I-Shin Shiah, Yue-Cune Chang, Tzu-Ju Lai, Kwua-Yun Wang, and Kuei-Ru Chou. 2004. 'Evaluation of an assertiveness training program on nursing and medical students' assertiveness, self-esteem, and interpersonal communication satisfaction.' *Nurse Education Today* 24 (8):656–665.

Lindström, Martin. 2006. 'Social capital and lack of belief in the possibility to influence one's own health: A population-based study.' *Scandinavian Journal of Public Health* 34 (1):69–75.

Linehan, Marsha M., Martin Bohus, and Thomas R. Lynch. 2007. 'Dialectical behavior therapy for pervasive emotion dysregulation.' *Handbook of Emotion Regulation* 1:581–605.

Linton, Steven J. 2013. 'A transdiagnostic approach to pain and emotion.' *Journal of Applied Biobehavioral Research* 18 (2):82–103.

Longden, E., A. Madill, and M.G. Waterman. 2012. 'Dissociation, trauma, and the role of lived experience: Toward a new conceptualization of voice hearing.' *Psychological Bulletin* 138 (1):28–76. doi:10.1037/a0025995.

Lynch, J.M. 2019. *Sense of safety: A whole person approach to distress.* PhD, Primary Care Clinical Unit, University of Queensland.

Lysaker, Paul H., Amanda M. Wickett, Neil Wilke, and John Lysaker. 2003. 'Narrative incoherence in schizophrenia: The absent agent-protagonist and the collapse of internal dialogue.' *American Journal of Psychotherapy* 57 (2):153–166.

Madhyastha, Tara M., Ellen L. Hamaker, and John M. Gottman. 2011. 'Investigating spousal influence using moment-to-moment affect data from marital conflict.' *Journal of Family Psychology* 25 (2):292–300. doi:10.1037/a0023028.

Marmot, Michael. 2005. 'Social determinants of health inequalities.' *The Lancet* 365 (9464):1099–1104.

Maslow, A.H. 1954. *Motivation and personality third edition.* Edited by R. Frager, J. Fadiman, C. McReynolds, and R. Cox. New York: Harper Collins Publishers.

McConnell, Kelly M., Kenneth I. Pargament, Christopher G. Ellison, and Kevin J. Flannelly. 2006. 'Examining the links between spiritual struggles and symptoms of psychopathology in a national sample.' *Journal of Clinical Psychology* 62 (12):1469–1484.

McDermid, Ann J., Gary B. Rollman, and Glenn A. McCain. 1996. 'Generalized hypervigilance in fibromyalgia: Evidence of perceptual amplification.' *PAIN®* 66 (2–3):133–144.

McGilchrist, Iain. 2019. *The master and his emissary: The divided brain and the making of the Western world.* London: Yale University Press.

Meares, Russell. 1986. 'On the ownership of thought: An approach to the origins of separation anxiety.' *Psychiatry* 49 (1):80–91.

Meares, Russell. 2000. *Intimacy and alienation: Memory, trauma and personal being.* New York: Routledge.

Meares, Russell. 2012. *A dissociation model of borderline personality disorder.* London: WW Norton & Company.

Middleton, Hugh. 2016. 'Flourishing and posttraumatic growth. An empirical take on ancient wisdoms.' *Health Care Analysis* 24 (2):133–147.

Mikulincer, M. 1995. 'Attachment style and the mental representation of the self.' *Journal of Personality and Social Psychology* 69 (6):1203–1215.

Milton, Abul, Mijanur Rahman, Sumaira Hussain, Charulata Jindal, Sushmita Choudhury, Shahnaz Akter, Shahana Ferdousi, Tafzila Mouly, John Hall, and Jimmy Efird. 2017. 'Trapped in statelessness: Rohingya refugees in Bangladesh.' *International Journal of Environmental Research and Public Health* 14 (942). https://www.mdpi.com/1660-4601/14/8/942#cite

Min, Meeyoung, Kathleen Farkas, Sonia Minnes, and Lynn T. Singer. 2007. 'Impact of childhood abuse and neglect on substance abuse and psychological distress in adulthood.' *Journal of Traumatic Stress* 20 (5):833–844.

Modell, Arnold. 2008. 'The agency of the self and the brain's illusions.' In *Psychological agency: Theory, practice, and culture*, edited by R. Frie, 35–49. Cambridge, MA: MIT Press.

Mount, Balfour. 1993. 'Whole person care: Beyond psychosocial and physical needs.' *American Journal of Hospice and Palliative Medicine* 10 (1):28–37.

Murray, Judith. 2015. *Understanding loss: A guide for caring for those facing adversity*. London: Routledge.

Nagoski, E. and A. Nagoski. 2020. *Burnout: The secret to unlocking the stress cycle*. New York, Ballantine Books.

Najavits, Lisa M., Robert J. Gallop, and Roger D. Weiss. 2006. 'Seeking safety therapy for adolescent girls with PTSD and substance use disorder: A randomized controlled trial.' *The Journal of Behavioral Health Services & Research* 33 (4):453–463.

Neff, Kristin. 2003. 'Self-compassion: An alternative conceptualization of a healthy attitude toward oneself.' *Self and Identity* 2 (2):85–101.

Neff, Kristin D., Kristin L. Kirkpatrick, and Stephanie S. Rude. 2007. 'Self-compassion and adaptive psychological functioning.' *Journal of Research in Personality* 41 (1):139–154.

Neimeyer, Robert A.. 1997. *Meaning reconstruction and the experience of chronic loss*. Edited by K.J. Doka, and J. Davidson, *Living with grief when illness is prolonged*. Bristol: Taylor & Francis.

Neimeyer, Robert A. 2001. *Meaning reconstruction & the experience of loss*. Washington, DC: American Psychological Association.

Norman, Kenneth A., Ehren Newman, Greg Detre, and Sean Polyn. 2006. 'How inhibitory oscillations can train neural networks and punish competitors.' *Neural Computation* 18 (7):1577–1610.

Norton, Peter J., and Debra A. Hope. 2001. 'Kernels of truth or distorted perceptions: Self and observer ratings of social anxiety and performance.' *Behavior Therapy* 32 (4):765–786.

O'Hanlon, Bill, and Bob Bertolino. 1998. *Even from a broken web: Brief, respectful solution-oriented therapy for sexual abuse and trauma*. New York: W.W. Norton and Co.

O'keeffe, Nikki, and Gopinath Ranjith. 2007. 'Depression, demoralisation or adjustment disorder? Understanding emotional distress in the severely medically ill.' *Clinical Medicine* 7 (5):478–481.

Origgi, Gloria. 2012. 'Epistemic injustice and epistemic trust.' *Social Epistemology* 26 (2):221–235.

Otter, Thomas. 2011. 'Has the financial crisis shattered citizens' trust in national and European governmental institutions?' In CEPS Working Document, Centre for European Policy Studies.

Park, Crystal L. 2013. 'The meaning making model: A framework for understanding meaning, spirituality, and stress-related growth in health psychology.' *European Health Psychologist* 15 (2):40–47.

Paulson, Sandra, ed. 2017. When there are no words: Repairing *early* Trauma and *neglect from the attachment period with* EMDR *therapy*. Bainbridge: Createspace Independent Publishing Platform.

Perry, B. 2020. *Staying close in the time of COVID-19 podcast*. https://www.the traumatherapistproject.com/podcast/bruce-perry-md-phd-staying-emotionally-close-in-the-time-of-covid-19/

Phillips, Maggie, and Claire Frederick. 1995. *Healing the divided self: Clinical and Ericksonian hypnotherapy for post-traumatic and dissociative conditions.* New York: WW Norton & Company.

Phillips III, Russell E., and Catherine H. Stein. 2007. 'God's will, God's punishment, or God's limitations? Religious coping strategies reported by young adults living with serious mental illness.' *Journal of Clinical Psychology* 63 (6):529–540.

Pols, Jeannette. 2006. 'Washing the citizen: Washing, cleanliness and citizenship in mental health care.' *Culture, Medicine and Psychiatry* 30 (1):77–104.

Porges, Stephen W., and Gregory F. Lewis. 2010. 'The polyvagal hypothesis: Common mechanisms mediating autonomic regulation, vocalizations and listening.' In *Handbook of mammalian vocalisation,* edited by S.M. Brudzynski, 255–264. London: Academic Press.

Posner, Michael I., Mary K. Rothbart, Brad E. Sheese, and Yiyuan Tang. 2007. 'The anterior cingulate gyrus and the mechanism of self-regulation.' *Cognitive, Affective, & Behavioral Neuroscience* 7 (4):391–395.

Preece, David A., Rodrigo Becerra, Ken Robinson, Justine Dandy, and Alfred Allan. 2018. 'Measuring emotion regulation ability across negative and positive emotions: The Perth Emotion Regulation Competency Inventory (PERCI).' *Personality and Individual Differences* 135:229–241.

Reeve, Joanne. 2010. 'Interpretive medicine: Supporting generalism in a changing primary care world.' *Occasional Paper Royal College of General Practitioners* 88:1–20.

Reeve, Joanne, M. Lloyd-Williams, and S. Payne. 2012. 'From personal challenge to technical fix: The risks of depersonalised care.' *Health & Social Care in the Community,* 20 (2):145–154.

Riquino, Michael R., Sarah E. Priddy, Matthew O. Howard, and Eric L. Garland. 2018. 'Emotion dysregulation as a transdiagnostic mechanism of opioid misuse and suicidality among chronic pain patients.' *Borderline Personality Disorder and Emotion Dysregulation* 5 (11). https://doi.org/10.1186/s40479-018-0088-6.

Ross, Catherine E., and John Mirowsky. 2009. 'Neighborhood disorder, subjective alienation, and distress.' *Journal of Health and Social Behavior* 50 (1):49–64.

Rothbart, Mary K., and M. Rosario Rueda. 2005. 'The development of effortful control.' In *Developing individuality in the human brain: A tribute to Michael I. Posner,* edited by E. Mayr, and S. Keele, 167–188. Washington, DC: American Psychological Association.

Rothbart, Mary K., Brad E. Sheese, M. Rosario Rueda, and Michael I. Posner. 2011. 'Developing mechanisms of self-regulation in early life.' *Emotion Review* 3 (2):207–213.

Ruffolo, Jessica S., Katharine A. Phillips, William Menard, Christina Fay, and Risa B. Weisberg. 2006. 'Comorbidity of body dysmorphic disorder and eating disorders: Severity of psychopathology and body image disturbance.' *International Journal of Eating Disorders* 39 (1):11–19.

Salter, Mary D. 1940. *An evaluation of adjustment based upon the concept of security.* University of Toronto Studies, Child Development Series.

Saunders, Rachel, Deborah Jacobvitz, Maria Zaccagnino, Lauren M. Beverung, and Nancy Hazen. 2011. 'Pathways to earned-security: The role of alternative support figures.' *Attachment & Human Development* 13 (4):403–420.

Scaer, Robert. 2014. *The body bears the burden: Trauma, dissociation, and disease.* New York: Routledge. Taylor and Francis Group.

Schore, Allan N., ed. 1994. *Affect regulation and the origin of the self.* New Jersey: Lawrence Erlbaum and Associates.

Schwartz, Richard C., and Robert R. Falconer. 2017. *Many minds, one self: Evidence for a radical shift in paradigm*. Oak Park, IL: Trailheads.

Schwartz, Richard C., and Martha Sweezy. 2019. *Internal family systems therapy*. New York: Guilford Publications.

Sebastian, Juliann G. 1985. 'Homelessness: A state of vulnerability.' *Family & Community Health: The Journal of Health Promotion & Maintenance* 8 (3):11–24. https://doi.org /10.1097/00003727-198511000-00003.

Seigel, Daniel, and Mary Hartzell. 2003. *Parenting from the inside out*. New York: Jeremy P. Tarcher.

Sen, Amartya. 1993. 'Capability and well-being.' In *The quality of life*, edited by M Nussbaum and Amartya Sen, 30–36. Oxford: Clarendon Press. https://oxford. universitypressscholarship.com/view/10.1093/0198287976.001.0001/acprof-9780198287971-chapter-5?print=pdf

Shonkoff, Jack P., Andrew S. Garner, Benjamin S. Siegel, Mary I. Dobbins, Marian F. Earls, Laura McGuinn, John Pascoe, David L Wood, and Committee on Psychosocial Aspects of Child, Family Health, Adoption Committee on Early Childhood, and Dependent Care. 2012. 'The lifelong effects of early childhood adversity and toxic stress.' *Pediatrics* 129 (1):e232–e246.

Siegel, D.J., ed. 2010. *Mindsight*. Oxford: One World.

Siegel, D.J. 2001. 'Toward an interpersonal neurobiology of the developing mind: Attachment relationships, "mindsight," and neural integration.' *Infant Mental Health Journal* 22 (1–2):67–94.

Siegel, Judith M. 1993. 'Companion animals: In sickness and in health.' *Journal of Social Issues* 49 (1):157–167.

Simmons, W. Kyle, Jason A. Avery, Joel C. Barcalow, Jerzy Bodurka, Wayne C. Drevets, and Patrick Bellgowan. 2013. 'Keeping the body in mind: Insula functional organization and functional connectivity integrate interoceptive, exteroceptive, and emotional awareness.' *Human Brain Mapping* 34 (11):2944–2958.

Skinner, Ellen A., and Melanie J. Zimmer-Gembeck. 2007. 'The development of coping.' *Annual Review of. Psychology* 58:119–144.

Sloan, Elise, Kate Hall, Richard Moulding, Shayden Bryce, Helen Mildred, and Petra K. Staiger. 2017. 'Emotion regulation as a transdiagnostic treatment construct across anxiety, depression, substance, eating and borderline personality disorders: A systematic review.' *Clinical Psychology Review* 57:141–163.

Sloan, Tracy, and Michael J. Telch. 2002. 'The effects of safety-seeking behavior and guided threat reappraisal on fear reduction during exposure: An experimental investigation.' *Behaviour Research and Therapy* 40 (3):235–251.

Somer, Eli. 2002. 'Maladaptive daydreaming: A qualitative inquiry.' *Journal of Contemporary Psychotherapy* 32 (2–3):197–212.

Somer, Eli, Liora Somer, and Daniela S. Jopp. 2016. 'Parallel lives: A phenomenological study of the lived experience of maladaptive daydreaming.' *Journal of Trauma & Dissociation* 17 (5):561–576.

Southwick, Steven M., George A. Bonanno, Ann S. Masten, Catherine Panter-Brick, and Rachel Yehuda. 2014. 'Resilience definitions, theory, and challenges: Interdisciplinary perspectives.' *European Journal of Psychotraumatology* 5 (1):25338. doi:10.3402/ejpt. v5.25338.

Speckhard, A., and N. Mufel. 2003. 'Universal responses to abortion? Attachment, Trauma, and grief responses in women following abortion.' *Journal of Prenatal and Perinatal Psychology*:3–37.

Spector, Paul E., Cary L. Cooper, Juan I. Sanchez, Michael. O'Driscoll, Kate Sparks, Peggy Bernin, Andre Büssing, Phil Dewe, Peter Hart, and Luo Lu. 2001. 'Do national levels of individualism and internal locus of control relate to well-being: An ecological level international study.' *Journal of Organizational Behavior: The International Journal of Industrial, Occupational and Organizational Psychology and Behavior* 22 (8):815–832.

Spertus, Ilyse L., Rachel Yehuda, Cheryl M. Wong, Sarah Halligan, and Stephanie V. Seremetis. 2003. 'Childhood emotional abuse and neglect as predictors of psychological and physical symptoms in women presenting to a primary care practice.' *Child Abuse & Neglect* 27 (11):1247–1258.

Spiegel, David, Roberto Lewis-Fernández, Ruth Lanius, Eric Vermetten, Daphne Simeon, and Matthew Friedman. 2013. 'Dissociative disorders in DSM-5.' *Annual Review of Clinical Psychology* 9:299–326.

Steger, Michael F. 2013. 'Experiencing meaning in life: Optimal functioning at the nexus of well-being, psychopathology, and spirituality.' In *The human quest for meaning*, edited by Paul T.P. Wong, 211–230. New York: Routledge.

Stein, Nancy L., and Tom Trabasso. 1992. 'The organisation of emotional experience: Creating links among emotion, thinking, language, and intentional action.' *Cognition & Emotion* 6 (3–4):225–244.

Stroebe, Margaret, and Henk Schut. 2010. 'The dual process model of coping with bereavement: A decade on.' *OMEGA-Journal of Death and Dying* 61 (4):273–289.

Talbot, Nancy L. 1996. 'Women sexually abused as children: The centrality of shame issues and treatment implications.' *Psychotherapy: Theory, Research, Practice, Training* 33 (1):11–18.

Tiggemann, Marika. 2011. 'Mental health risks of self-objectification: A review of the empirical evidence for disordered eating, depressed mood, and sexual dysfunction.' In *Self-objectification in women: Causes, consequences, and counteractions*, edited by R.M. Calogero, S. Tantleff-Dunn, and J.K. Thompson, 139–159. Washington, DC: American Psychological Association.

Tomasdottir, Margret Olafia, Johann Agust Sigurdsson, Halfdan Petursson, Anna Luise Kirkengen, Tom Ivar Lund Nilsen, Irene Hetlevik, and Linn Getz. 2016. 'Does "existential unease" predict adult multimorbidity? Analytical cohort study on embodiment based on the Norwegian HUNT population.' *BMJ Open* 6 (11):e012602. doi:10.1136/bmjopen-2016-012602.

Toomey, Brian, and Bruce Ecker. 2007. 'Of neurons and knowings: Constructivism, coherence psychology, and their neurodynamic substrates.' *Journal of Constructivist Psychology* 20 (3):201–245.

Vaitl, Dieter, Niels Birbaumer, John Gruzelier, Graham A. Jamieson, Boris Kotchoubey, Andrea Kübler, Dietrich Lehmann, Wolfgang H.R. Miltner, Ulrich Ott, and Peter Pütz. 2005. 'Psychobiology of altered states of consciousness.' *Psychological Bulletin* 131 (1):98–127.

Vandenbosch, Laura, and Johanna M.F. van Oosten. 2017. 'The relationship between online pornography and the sexual objectification of women: The attenuating role of porn literacy education.' *Journal of Communication* 67 (6):1015–1036.

Van der Kolk, Bessel A., and Alexander C. McFarlane. 2012. *Traumatic stress: The effects of overwhelming experience on mind, body, and society*. New York: The Guilford Press.

Vanderveren, Elien, Patricia Bijttebier, and Dirk Hermans. 2019. 'Autobiographical memory coherence and specificity: Examining their reciprocal relation and their associations with internalizing symptoms and rumination.' *Behaviour Research and Therapy* 116:30–35.

Van Praag, Herman M., Edo Ronald de Kloet, and Jim Van Os. 2004. *Stress, the brain and depression*. Cambridge: Cambridge University Press.

Venta, Amanda, Carla Sharp, Yael Shmueli-Goetz, and Elizabeth Newlin. 2015. 'An evaluation of the construct of earned security in adolescents: Evidence from an inpatient sample.' *Bulletin of the Menninger Clinic* 79 (1):41–69.

Waldfogel, Shimon. 1997. 'Spirituality in medicine.' *Primary Care: Clinics in Office Practice* 24 (4):963–976.

Walker, Shelley, Meredith Temple-Smith, Peter Higgs, and Lena Sanci. 2015. '"It's always just there in your face": Young people's views on porn.' *Sexual Health* 12 (3):200–206.

Wallace, Rodrick, and Deborah Wallace. 1997. 'Socioeconomic determinants of health: Community marginalisation and the diffusion of disease and disorder in the United States.' *BMJ: British Medical Journal* 314:1341. https://doi.org/10.1136/bmj.314.70 90.1341.

Walsh, Froma. 2015. *Strengthening family resilience*. New York: Guilford Publications.

Weine, Stevan Merill, Scott Langenecker, and Aliriza Arenliu. 2018. 'Global mental health and the national institute of mental health research domain criteria.' *International Journal of Social Psychiatry* 64 (5):436–442.

Wensing, Michel, Glyn Elwyn, Adrian Edwards, Eric Vingerhoets, and Richard Grol. 2002. 'Deconstructing patient centred communication and uncovering shared decision making: An observational study.' *BMC Medical Informatics and Decision Making* 2 (2). https://doi.org/10.1186/1472-6947-2-2.

Westerman, Michael A. 2007. 'Integrating the parts of the biopsychosocial model.' *Philosophy, Psychiatry, & Psychology* 14 (4):321–326.

Whiting, Jason B., Douglas B. Smith, Megan Oka, and Gunnur Karakurt. 2012. 'Safety in intimate partnerships: The role of appraisals and threat.' *Journal of Family Violence* 27 (4):313–320.

Williams, Fiona, and Penelope Hasking. 2010. 'Emotion regulation, coping and alcohol use as moderators in the relationship between non-suicidal self-injury and psychological distress.' *Prevention Science* 11 (1):33–41.

Woby, Steve R., Martin Urmston, and Paul J. Watson. 2007. 'Self-Efficacy mediates the relation between pain-related fear and outcome in chronic low back pain patients.' *European Journal of Pain* 11 (7):711–718.

Wright, Margaret O'Dougherty, Emily Crawford, and Darren Del Castillo. 2009. 'Childhood emotional maltreatment and later psychological distress among college students: The mediating role of maladaptive schemas.' *Child Abuse & Neglect* 33 (1):59–68.

10 *Sense of safety*

A paradigm shift that is sorely needed – accompanying Humpty and his community towards wholeness

- Generalist, transdisciplinary and indigenous ways of knowing can reveal new paradigm shifting ways of seeing wellbeing
- Translation in the real world will be difficult, but *sense of safety* is sorely needed in health and beyond
- Ways forward will involve a change in how we see the whole person, their experience of threat and safety and the dynamics that produce wellbeing

The thesis developed in this book is that generalist and transdisciplinary philosophy and practice mandate attending widely to the person, to threat, distress, healing, comfort, recovery and now to *sense of safety* as part of whole person care. Just like the Bowerbird, these approaches to research and practice gather fragments into patterns and see the complex whole as more than the sum of the parts. Generalist and transdisciplinary philosophy, alongside indigenous ways of knowing, offer something more than the 'body parts approach' (Hunter 1999). Instead, they value a relational, 'mind-heart connection' kind of listening (Atkinson 2002, 19). They tune in to each embodied person within their relationships, meaning and environment, including connection to community and country. The wide transdisciplinary literature referenced throughout this book gives scientific insights into the truly personalised interconnected physicality of these ancient wisdoms.

As well as transdisciplinary literature and generalist clinical experience, stakeholders and academics (*participants*) were asked to comment on the research as it developed. They were asked whether the concept of *sense of safety* that had developed made sense to them. Broad themes of participant feedback were that it was *out of the comfort zone*, would have *translation concerns*, and yet they *spontaneously applied* the concept to their own lives and practice, described it as *potentially useful, common sense* (ia) and *sorely needed* (gp). This feedback is integrated throughout this final discussion.

Sense of safety is a blueprint for a shared language. This language is Humpty's native tongue and acts as an ancient trade language – an embodied pattern that preceded and transcends disciplinary barriers. *Sense of safety* is also common sense;

it is ordinary and simple but not simplistic. It is a return to first principles that can disrupt silos with respect and connection. It is a deep communal need and a cross-cultural experience. As already established, it is a 'metaneed' (Maslow 1954), a fundamental building block for growth and wellbeing.

Sense of safety is a call to return to basic needs of personhood. It clearly includes relationships, meaning, context and life story as part of the multiple interconnected domains and dynamics that build safety. The concept of *sense of safety* names first principles and dynamics that can facilitate safety across the wider community and culture (including policies and practices). It can be built across the community – in friendships, family, work, learning and health. *Sense of safety* intentionally enfranchises indigenous ways of knowing, as well as non-academic forms of knowing such as intuition, art, music, spirituality and storytelling. Seeing people as complex beings widens the possibilities for healing. *Sense of safety* aligns with those who remind that 'plain old caring [has] sustained the human species for millennia' (Allen 2013, xxiii). It is a reminder of ordinary priorities for humane care that can get side-lined by biotechnological reductionist, theoretical sociological, professionalised or bureaucratised approaches to health. Rather than the domain of narrow professional guilds or pharmaceutical research companies, *sense of safety* could become communally understood as an ordinary pathway to wellbeing.

Healing can be described as 'the phenomenon of people becoming increasingly conscious of their own needs in multiple domains of their individual and collective existence, and an acknowledgement that these needs were unmet' (Atkinson 2002, 189). Appraising *sense of safety* could help us to identify and meet these needs of the whole embodied person within community.

'Sense of safety' is an ordinary phrase, part of Humpty's native tongue, that naturally integrates the physicality of the senses with integrative, whole person sense-making. It offers a way for both practitioner and Humpty to tune in to their own inherent appraisals of threat and capacity to cope with that threat. It is collaborative; it is incomplete without Humpty (and the practitioner) noticing and naming their integrative 'sense of' the situation. *Sense of safety* could protect us from fragmentated, individualised, de-personalised and spuriously precise ways of conceptualising wellbeing and the process of healing.

Out of the comfort zone: Can the King's Men learn a new language?

Current privileging of reductionist evidence and inherent fragmentation of disciplinary jargon dialects prevent the King's Men being able to 'put Humpty together again'. There are inherent limitations in biomedical and psychiatric approaches to personhood (Dowrick 2017). Instead of whole-hearted attending, Humpty is classified and labelled with nouns of disorder in ways that can prevent him from being seen. Even gathering of biopsychosocial fragments of knowledge, trans-diagnostic frameworks or mixed-methods research is not enough. Continuing to use the 'body parts' approaches to diagnosis means the fundamental difficulty of integrating knowledge across disciplines cannot be addressed. Any attempt to unify these silos requires access to knowledge stored inside institutional departmental structures, epistemic cultures and jargon-filled language that do not value or understand integrative approaches to knowledge. For the generalist, these fragmented approaches to the whole person are inadequate.

The concept of *sense of safety* aligns with those who call for an end to the 'out of date' 'disease era' with its attendant 'undertreatment, overtreatment, or mistreatment' (Tinetti and Fried 2004, 179). Experienced trauma therapist Richard Kluft says 'you violate a patient's dignity if you treat them with a theory that is inadequate – have the humility to remain confused' (Kluft 2015). Therefore, clinicians are ethically bound to not be satisfied with reductionist biomedical or sociological ways of seeing (Kirkengen and Thornquist 2012) and instead to sit in the confusion of an uncertainty of complexity. Generalists see a shift in paradigm as a moral imperative (Kirkengen and Thornquist 2012). Ian McWhinney again offers wisdom. He suggests:

> Reforming our clinical method has at its deepest level a moral purpose: a restoration of the balance between thinking and feeling, and a sharing of the enormous power modern technology has given us.
>
> (McWhinney et al. 1995)

Participants who gave feedback on the concept of *sense of safety* spontaneously compared *sense of safety* to the biopsychosocial approach. They called the biopsychosocial approach as it is currently used 'tokenism' (gp) and 'a kind of tick-boxy thing which does not do justice to what it was originally meant to be – even when it is done well' (mhc-a). They could see the scientific inadequacy of the status quo – 'we are taught a very old-fashioned way of thinking' (gp). They could also see the paradigm shift inherent in the concept of *sense of safety*, saying 'what you are talking about is a paradigm shift' (gp) and describing it as a 'complete reframing of the way we think about people and their context' (gp). One GP confessed: 'I think you are on to something, and it's something that needs to be shared. It is our job, but we haven't been taught well how to do it' (gp). Another signalled her concern about the paradigm shift, calling it courageous: 'it's very courageous. It's exactly what we need – a change in how we think about distress' (gp). This insightful feedback is heartening and also reinforces the reality of the inherent shift in paradigm: even though some participants saw it as 'common sense' (ia), it remains *out of the comfort zone* for the medical and wider community.

Translation concerns: A paradigm shift may be too difficult to deliver

In the real world, having a *sorely needed* and *common-sense* idea may not be enough. Getting papers published that do not align with a siloed linear research process or having reflective transdisciplinary collaboration funded is very difficult given the current positivist conceptualisation of 'science' or original 'evidence'. In a world driven by pharma, disease focus and productivity, who funds whole person approaches that empower but do not intend to sell a product?

Fragmentation is as normal as entropy; unity requires intentional input of energy. It requires champions and change of heart. Whose job is it in the community to gather knowledge and watch for patterns? Whose job is it to return us to first principles and champion new mindsets? In order for *sense of safety* to become part of ordinary care in our communities, we may need a shift away from the disciplinary professions towards valuing (and funding) transdisciplinary and generalist research and practice.

As discussed in Chapter Two, there are longstanding difficulties in attending to the whole person. Despite respect as an Aboriginal leader, tireless work advocating for holistic approaches to health for his people and a very evident inadequacy of the current approach, the late Puggy (Arnold) Hunter described difficulty creating paradigm change:

> We've been saying the same things for many years and no one hears. So I always think, gee you white fellas must have a really bad hearing problem as well because you don't seem to hear us very well because we haven't been saying anything different.
>
> (Hunter 2001)

Challenging the dominant biomedical paradigm from within, involves a shift from hierarchical disciplinary knowledge structures to transdisciplinary approaches. This shifts attention to knowledge that is necessarily on the border, a position on the edge of disciplines that means a loss of legitimacy and influence that can hamper translation. As Polk notes:

> Transdisciplinary processes are homeless. If they are based on joint ownership and decision making between research and practice, then they belong nowhere … they lack legitimacy outside their sphere of immediate practitioners. This lack of belonging and legitimacy has serious consequences for the ability of transdisciplinary research to contribute to sustainability in a wider sense.
>
> (Polk 2014, 450)

Another limitation – resistance within a profession to new reflective ways of seeing – is defined by Schon:

> Many practitioners, locked into a view of themselves as technical experts, find nothing in the world of practice to occasion reflection. They have become too skilful at techniques of selective inattention, junk categories, and situational control, techniques which they use to preserve the constancy of their knowledge-in-practice. For them, uncertainty is a threat; its admission is a sign of weakness. Others, more inclined toward and adept at reflection-in-action,

nevertheless feel profoundly uneasy because they cannot say what they know how to do, cannot justify its quality and rigor.

(Schön 1995, 69)

Participants, while confirming the concept of *sense of safety*'s usefulness, also bemoaned the difficulties it would face in translation: 'I think it's absolutely right and trying to get it through to people who most need to hear it, I think could be really challenging' (mhc). They spoke from experience within medical schools, saying: 'I think it is going to make a huge difference ... it's a fabulous idea ... But it's just how do you embed it?' (ia).

Is *sense of safety* another way to pathologise or a healing-oriented paradigm shift?

There were also participants who questioned whether the term *sense of safety* was merely another way to pathologise or medicalise people. A senior academic GP summarised these concerns: 'life is not about safety – challenges require that you feel unsafe a lot of the time – the word safety does not have the right feeling' (mhc-a). Some questioned whether it was even possible to feel safe, whether some people had ever felt safe and whether instead it was a quest, a direction to travel. One mental health clinician suggested 'balancing movement between safety and challenge – both are necessary for being whole' (mhc). Others could see its potential to align with other movements towards safety, saying it was 'cultural safety for everybody' (gp).

Psychological researchers question any framework that encourages 'a sense of virtuous but impotent victimhood' (Haslam 2016, 1), which they see can occur if concepts extend 'outward to capture qualitatively new phenomena and downward to capture quantitatively less extreme phenomena' (Haslam 2016, 1). This is one of the risks in wide generalist frameworks that seek to facilitate early intervention. *Sense of safety* has intentionally sought to increase the breadth and depth of awareness of distress, which could mean a widening of the pathologising medical gaze. It has, however, intentionally directed attention towards the goal of healing and the dynamics that build *sense of safety*. It is healing-centred or healing-oriented. It draws attention to resources and strengths that build *sense of safety* in a way that does not pathologise. *Sense of safety* involves both 'comfort' and 'courage'. It involves movement towards engagement and connection rather than escape and disconnection.

Sense of safety also normalises experiences that are currently pathologised. Emotions, for example, are often seen as troublesome moods (or mood disorders) rather than considered sensory information and communication, while defences are often pathologised as substance abuse or compulsive disorders rather than seen as logical distress reduction behaviours. Attending to threat and seeking to understand it, from whatever internal or external cause, can make seemingly disordered responses make sense.

Sense of safety also demythologises healing and places it within reach of those who have no contact with professional healers. The dynamics of *respectful connection* and *capable engagement* offer ordinary understandable directions of travel that build *sense of safety* across the community. The internal dynamics of *calm sense-making, broad awareness* and *owning yourself* help Humpty learn how to make sense of his world. *Sense of safety* positions healing within relationships and shifts responsibility for healing away from individualised 'dis-ease' towards systemic causes of loss of *sense of safety* in the environment, social climate and relationships. These shifts in how the community sees wellbeing are a shift away from naming *nouns of disorder* (in behaviour and symptoms), towards wider *verbs of wellbeing* – patterns that can build *sense of safety*.

Sense of safety: Sorely needed in health and beyond

As has been argued extensively throughout this book and the underlying doctoral research it is built on, *sense of safety* is a legitimate integrative way to see the whole person; it aligns with generalist, transdisciplinary and indigenous ways of seeing the whole. It is physiologically grounded and integrates a wide, relevant transdisciplinary literature. It enfranchises the voice, sensations and sense-making of the sufferer. It is a part of Humpty's ancient embodied native tongue – and therefore has the potential to be readily understood by the community. As one participant responded:

> Overall, I think the greatest strength of the approach you are describing in the simplest idea at its core – that people in primary care are often bothered by distress that emerges from their lives in all of their complexity and that this can be missed or misconstrued by conventional approaches to the physician-patient interaction. ... the approach you are developing has great potential. (mhc-a)

Just as the patient who described her *sense of safety* as being 'like a deep breath', clinicians seemed to readily understand the physicality and relevance of this concept and apply it to their own work:

> I think that concept of making the person safe, in this moment, that's something that really resonates with me because it's so much of it is about how you engage with that person. And if you engage with them the right way, you get completely different outcomes. (gp)

They also commented on the validity of the concept saying: 'Your paper is quite compelling and exquisitely researched. It describes a fundamental human need that clearly intersects with the daily work of physicians' (gp-a). They saw it as evidence-based and fulfilling a practical need:

> it is straightforward, comes from an evidentiary base ... comes from a thoughtful review of the literature, translates into a pragmatic attitudinal position for the clinician which then opens up the possibility of some fairly

pragmatic straightforward sort of things – you empower clinicians around a group of patients that they really don't know what to do with. (mhc-a)

This framework therefore has a mandate from stakeholders (including end-users) and academics; it has the potential to direct clinical reasoning and goal setting, influence research priorities and offer a way to frame self-care for practitioners. A number of non-medical stakeholders expressed their belief that their own profession would benefit from the concept of *sense of safety*. A new mindset that facilitates *sense of safety* is not only *sorely needed*, it is a legitimate way to frame wellbeing for each person that resonates in health and beyond, to the whole community.

Practical directions: Walking with Humpty towards health

Throughout this book, a number of maps have been used to outline the key paradigm shifts. These have included those that bring awareness to the types of knowledge that are part of the whole; those that bring attention to the processes that build, protect and reveal *sense of safety*; those that name the purposes of the senses and those that define the goals of therapeutic and communal movement towards health.

These maps could guide the practical steps of walking with Humpty towards wellbeing. They could be applied within the consultation room or translated into wider community systems, across cultures and tribes, through policy direction into schools and workplaces. They could be used to justify closer collaboration across aspects of the whole from environment to housing, social services, workplace, education and health. They could be used to shift the language from disease, disorder or trauma towards the goal of building *sense of safety* in every setting, within the person, their family and their community. This shift will entail new value being placed on generalist skills of seeing the whole person and transdisciplinary research processes. It will include a new awareness of the whole person experience of threat, the importance of the senses, dynamics of change and new communal strength-based goals of wellbeing.

Valuing generalist, transdisciplinary and indigenous ways of seeing the whole

This practical step is a paradigm shift. It would mean a disruption of the status quo. It would require policy, research funding and health funding changes. Although these changes have been advocated for internationally for decades, there are forces that are resistant to change (Greenhalgh 2008, Gunn et al. 2008). The Declaration of Alma Ata (WHO 1978), the Declaration of Astana (Ghebreyesus et al. 2018) and the Ottawa Charter require generalist approaches to the whole person.

There are calls, therefore, for primary care to be a 'political rather than a palliative force' (Gibbs 2015, 154), driving change in the conceptualisation of wellbeing in our communities and resisting siloed reductionist ways of seeing the whole. Generalists call for a renewed valuing of generalist time and whole person priorities, saying 'thick detailed descriptions ... require time to collect' (Kirkengen 2005, 21). This is especially relevant in the context of chronic illness: 'the most relevant examination to set up for the enigmatic patient is an extended consultation giving room for complete history taking' (Getz 1999, 71).

The generalist, transdisciplinary and indigenous ways of knowing championed in this book have the potential to integrate diverse and ground-breaking research into whole person care. The *whole person knowledge map* (Figure 10.1) and *sense of safety domains* (Figure 10.2) remind us of the breadth of knowledge that should be considered in research and practice when caring for the whole person. They remind of the importance of both objective *biomedical* and subjective, sensory, *biographical* knowledge. They remind of the importance of meaning, sense of self, relationships, and communal environment. They offer an answer to Centor's (2007, 59) challenge outlined in the author statement 'to be a great physician you must understand the whole story ... gather the history at appropriate depth'. These maps suggest an answer to the questions 'what is that whole story?' and 'what is an appropriate depth?'

These maps could prompt new generalist and transdisciplinary standards defining what research has genuinely considered the whole person. At present, generalist approaches to knowledge are not respected within the research community that highly values repeatable reductionist 'original data'. A Norwegian think tank is already calling for new approaches to research that contribute to a 'deeper and more comprehensive theoretical framework for human sickness and health than the biomedical approach currently allows for' (Getz, Luise Kirkengen, and Hetlevik 2008, 65). They note that generalist priorities may not be considered

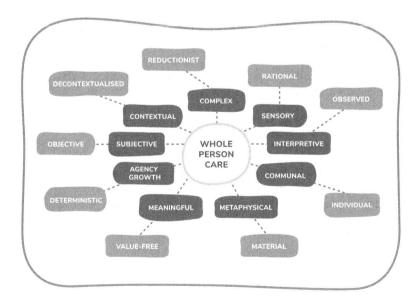

Figure 10.1 Whole person knowledge map.

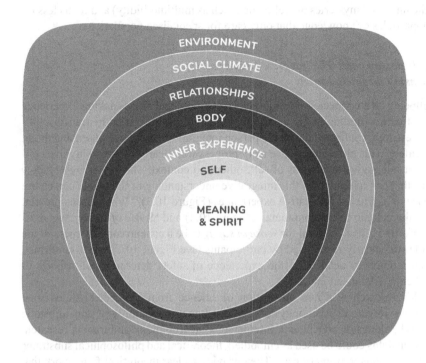

Figure 10.2 Sense of safety whole person domains.

'"researchable" with reference to mainstream study designs and methodologies' (Getz, Luise Kirkengen, and Hetlevik 2008, 65). They call for academic acknowledgement of the original research inherent in 'creative and skilled reflection' (Getz, Luise Kirkengen, and Hetlevik 2008, 66).

Valuing generalist and transdisciplinary ways of seeing the whole might mean that research that studied only a part of the whole would need to acknowledge the areas of the whole they did not consider. This would be a kind of product warning – outlining the limitations of their work for those seeking to use it in a generalist or primary care setting. Research journals and academic structures would also need to shift to see the integrative wisdom of the generalist, their relational skills, their clear healing focus and their sensitivity to broad sources of information that may be useful to the wider community. This would mean practical changes – the generalist needs to refer to wide sources of information (not just assumed linear knowledge formation) – and so needs more room for references! The generalist values gathering words and language as data and values experiential wisdom – so in-text quotations and named researcher citation styles may become more normal in health literature. International collaboration on this project may lead to new research structures that encourage reflective wisdom and transdisciplinary collaborative work, while discouraging projects that seek new data without overarching purpose. These endeavours would prioritise the *gestalt* underlying some of the unsolved mysteries of wellbeing (such as multimorbidity) and focus less on nanoparticles of knowledge that only care for specialised populations.

Whole person care: The integrated experience of sensing threat and safety

Wellbeing as a connected physiological, relational and sense-making experience is another key finding of this research. Stakeholders, backed up by transdisciplinary research, confirmed the whole person integrative experience of sensing threat and safety. This physiological, sensory process was clearly shown to involve concurrent integrative awareness of self, other and context. The key *sense of safety* maps that can remind us of this integrative understanding of the whole person are '*Sense of safety*: an integrative experience' (Figure 10.3), 'What senses protect: from the cellular to the communal' (Figure 10.4) and '*Sense of safety dynamics*' (Figure 10.5). The potential for *sense of safety* to be a concurrent awareness of the whole was clearly recognised by participants (see Figure 10.3) and is confirmed by an indigenous academic: 'the experience of safety determines all aspects of wellbeing' (Atkinson 2002, 45).

This research is a rare integration of science from biomedical fields such as stress research, psychophysiology, psychoneuroimmunology and allostatic research, alongside attachment, interpersonal neurobiology and trauma research. These insights could be used as embodied, theoretical and philosophical substrates for innovations in primary care. They provide a clear theoretical framework that

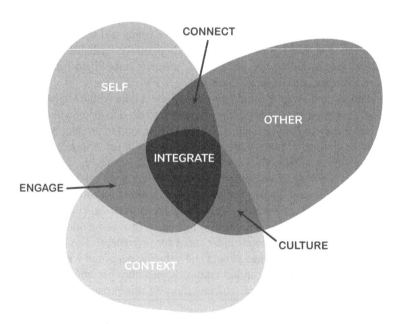

Figure 10.3 Sense of safety: an integrative experience.

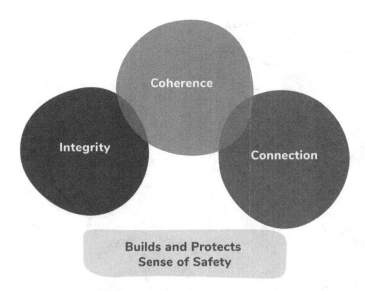

Figure 10.4 What senses protect: from the cellular to the communal.

defines not only the breadth but also the depth of knowing that is whole person care. These insights are grounded in physiological positivist *evidence* and post-positivist *experience* and transdisciplinary generalist *wisdom*. They could lead to new ways for Humpty to notice his own wellbeing and a renewed interest in self-rated health. The *sense of safety* concept could be translated into new outcome measures, self-care tools, clinical reasoning frameworks and ways to understand intuitive clinical appraisal skills. It can lead to innovative ways to promote well-being, such as were used for health workers during the time of COVID-19 (see Appendix II). It could also lead to new questions and answers in areas of health that are constrained by current approaches, for example, mood disorders, suici-dality, medically unexplained symptoms, chronic pain, somatisation and avoidant anxiety and addictive behaviours.

Attending to subjective experience is intentionally built into the concept of *sense of safety*. It includes the inherent internal sensing, perceiving and meaning-making that are part of being a person encountering life. 'Sense of' enfranchises perception, attention, sensation, sense of self and meaning as important aspects of wellbeing. It enfranchises Humpty's voice in his native tongue. It also enfran-chises the skills of a practitioner with honed perception and integrative wisdom, not just technical knowledge. These subjective experiences get easily ignored in positivist scientific frameworks; they also often get minimised as illogical or unre-liable. The *sense of safety* approach to sensation sees it as purposeful and integra-tive. As depicted in Figure 10.4, the first principle that sensation purposefully protects *integrity*, *connection* and *coherence* is a key concept. Sensation helps

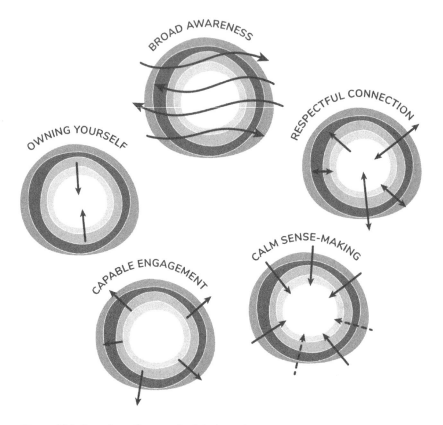

Figure 10.5 Overview of *sense of safety dynamics.*

both clinician and practitioner make sense of patterns of behaviour, symptoms, cellular homeostasis, relationship dynamics and communal rituals. *Sense of safety* offers a link between subjective and objective information that could encourage practitioners (and their teachers) to attend to and make sense of their own and Humpty's experience.

Sense of safety can also orient the practitioner to their own skills of awareness in the consultation (and in their own lives), as well as give a clear framework for questions that might be relevant for health. Being aware of self, other and context in every encounter and awareness of the purposes of sensation may lead to clear lines of questioning. For example, the question 'Is there anyone in your world who makes you feel confused, invaded or disconnected?' can be used to screen for unsafe relationships. The broad *sense of safety dynamics* (See Figure 10.5) also offer a direction of travel within the consultation and could enable patients to name their own directions of growth. Making sure each consultation increases the person's sense of *capable engagement, respectful connection* and capacity to for *owning themselves* could shift how treatment decision-making is enacted. Noticing the subtle ways that *broad awareness* has been lost in descriptions of an event or person may give direction to the next questions and skill training within a consultation. Facilitating *calm sense-making* could become a key named therapeutic process. As a first principle, *sense of safety* repeatedly reminds practitioners to attend to the integrated whole person, gives a coherent understanding of the whole person purpose of sensing and the *sense of safety dynamics* that build, protect and reveal *sense of safety*.

Building sense of safety: A strengths-based and dynamic approach to wellbeing

Sense of safety also offers a shared language focused on dynamic processes of growth towards *sense of safety*. This includes the concept of *verbs of wellbeing* discussed in Chapter Eight, the *sense of safety dynamics* (Figure 10.5) discussed in detail in Chapter Nine, 'Reframing Maslow: *sense of safety whole person goals*' (Figure 10.6) outlined in the 'Strengths-based trauma-informed *sense of safety goals of care*' (Figure 10.7). These adaptations of key frameworks (trauma-informed care and Maslow's hierarchy of needs) are built on the transdisciplinary

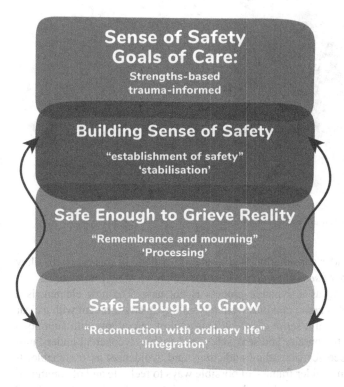

Figure 10.6 Trauma-informed and strengths-based *sense of safety goals of care*.

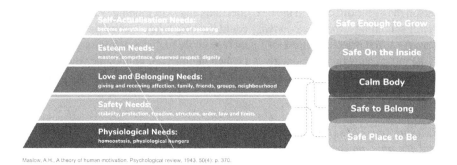

Maslow, A.H., A theory of human motivation. Psychological review, 1943. 50(4): p. 370.

Figure 10.7 Reframing Maslow: *sense of safety whole person goals.*

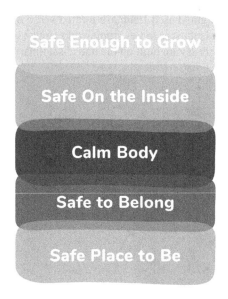

Figure 10.8 Sense of safety whole person goals.

literature, stakeholder consultation, and academic critique of this research. They embed the concept of *sense of safety* within robust pre-existing frameworks.

Seeing wellbeing as a dynamic process is not new. The new element is a grounding in *whole person domains* from physiology to environment with a clear direction or goal of care: *sense of safety*. This goal of care aligns with Humpty's pre-existing need to appraise and seek safety and enables a coherent understanding of coping processes (including addictions and avoidance) as reasonable. It places them within a wider frame – of possible ways to feel safe and of communal contributions to that safety. These dynamics are intrapsychic, interpersonal and embodied and can therefore be seen as patterns that link physiology, relationships, environment and life story.

The *sense of safety dynamics* clearly describe overarching goals and patterns to be attended to, appraised and enhanced in each consultation. They are broad directions of travel. Linking them with trauma-informed care principles (as in Figure 10.6) provides a safe process of care that includes a movement between building *sense of safety*, feeling *safe enough to grieve reality* and being *safe enough to grow* at each stage prioritising *sense of safety*.

Noticing the links with Maslow's hierarchy of needs (as in Figure 10.7) helps to see *sense of safety* as a meta-need across the *whole person domains*: environment (*safe place to be*), relationships and social climate (*safe to belong*), body (*calm body*), inner experience and sense of self (*safe on the inside*) and spirit/ meaning (*safe enough to grow*).

Again, as can be seen in Figure 10.8, physiological reality (calm body) is placed centrally, interacting externally with context and relationships and internally with inner experiences and meaning. Biology and biography and their interconnections are integrated in this whole person approach. These ways of understanding wellbeing clearly direct any therapeutic or communal policy processes towards the central goal of building *sense of safety* across all of the *whole person domains*.

Sense of safety dynamics can be observed and taught. They can be implemented across the community as clear goals of care. They are described in language that is part of Humpty's native tongue, making them ordinary and potentially teachable from the family, to the classroom, to the boardroom. *Sense of safety* is clearly linked to growth, to dynamic responses to life in all its richness, to awareness of strengths and resources, to new priorities, skills and goals. This shift away from medicalised diagnosis of disorder or symptoms (nouns), towards dynamics of growth that build *sense of safety* (verbs) is a foundation of the *sense of safety* approach to the whole person.

Conclusion

The attempt to think widely about the 'whole' person in the midst of an unfathomable amount of literature raises concerns that major areas of enquiry will be ignored or those that are attended to will be not accounted for in a complete way. The breadth of this topic and the complexity of each human story means that this way of seeing is necessarily incomplete and provisional and therefore open to critique. And yet it is important. It offers a shared language that integrates the complex interplay of influences on a person in distress. It offers new research at the interface of social and biomedical sciences (McDade 2008), asking new questions about how we approach the whole person.

In reflecting on the purpose of this book, I would dare to say that all mature practitioners become transdisciplinary. As these 'beleaguered defenders of holism' (Sadler 2005, 7) seek to serve their community, they are willing to learn from beyond their own 'discipline of origin'. Stakeholders revealed this openness to the whole when they intuitively endorsed the common sense of *sense of safety* as an essential for healing. The beautiful simplicity of this concept is revealed in experienced advice to trauma clinicians: 'if the therapist orients himself according to the issue of safety, the therapeutic task can become relatively simple' (Rappoport 1997, 261).

Reflective healer Henri Nouwen reminds us of the centrality of storytelling, relationship and hospitality in healing that seems to describe a place where both healer and patient experience *sense of safety*:

> Healers are hosts who patiently and carefully listen to the story of the suffering strangers. Patients are guests who rediscover their selves by telling their story to the one who offers them a place to stay. In the telling of their stories, strangers befriend not only their host, but also their own past.
>
> (Henri Nouwen 1975 in Balint 1993, 93)

> What does hospitality as a healing power require? It requires first of all that the host feel at home in his own house, and secondly that he create a free and fearless place for the unexpected visitor
>
> (Nouwen 1979, 81)

The *sense of safety* approach is focused on this free and fearless kind of healing. In this book, I propose the concept of *sense of safety* as a coherent healing-oriented way to approach people who are distressed. This synthesis of complex science, stakeholder consultation and academic critique is so grounded in transdisciplinary science and experience that it is considered to be at once *common-sense* and a *sense of safety*. It is ordinary language that gathers and integrates and makes sense. It is a physiologically legitimate and relationally authentic concept that could unify, transform and empower everyday healing. It is intentionally broad and inclusive as well as sensory and dynamic, countering current fragmenting classifications that do not make space for growth and healing. This concept of *sense of safety* includes not just a sense of *comfort*, but also a sense of capacity or *courage* to engage with life and grow. It is designed to include the voice (and sense) of the distressed in their own wellbeing and be applicable to all people, including those who care for the distressed in their worlds.

I end with an endorsement and a plea from an indigenous academic stakeholder during consultation about *sense of safety*:

> My gut reaction is great, good, something is happening, There's a sense of excitement in what you're doing and a sense of sadness because we critically need workers who can engage with small kids who come into the education system who are already in heightened sense of lack of safety, who act out and immediately they're suspended, expelled, and then they're moving straight down to juvenile detention, adult prison, we haven't got it … So, what you are doing is unpacking all of this and putting it into a package. (ia)

Perhaps *sense of safety* provides us (you, the reader and I) with a new mindset and heart attitude toward the whole person. It offers a map (*sense of safety domains*), a direction of travel (*sense of safety whole person goals*), and a collaborative way to journey there (*sense of safety dynamics*). This map, journey and direction of travel can guide our Bowerbird foraging and can refine our understanding of Humpty's native tongue as we search for the beauty and healing in the whole. *Sense of safety* domains and dynamics are a robust combination of content and process that can help us to step forward towards distress with a clear sense of how wide we have to look and what dynamics will help to bring healing in our communities worldwide.

References

Allen, J.G. 2013. *Restoring mentalizing in attachment relationships: Treating trauma with plain old therapy*. Washington: American Psychiatric Publishing.

Atkinson, J. 2002. *Trauma trails: Recreating songlines. The transgenerational effects of trauma in Indigenous Australia*. Melbourne: Spinifex Press.

Balint, E., ed. 1993. *The doctor, the patient and the group: Balint revisited*. London: Routledge.

Centor, Robert M. 2007. 'To be a great physician, you must understand the whole story.' *Medscape General Medicine* 9 (1):59.

Dowrick, Christopher. 2017. *Person-centred primary care: Searching for the self*. London: Routledge.

Getz, Linn. 1999. '"Unexplainable" medical histories and childhood sexual abuse: New doctoral thesis tells you how to investigate the links.' *Scandinavian Journal of Primary Health Care* 17 (2):68–71.

Getz, Linn, Anna Luise Kirkengen, and Irene Hetlevik. 2008. 'Too much doing and too little thinking in medical science!' *Scandinavian Journal of Primary Health Care* 26 (2):65–66.

Ghebreyesus, Tedros Adhanom, Henrietta Fore, Yelzhan Birtanov, and Zsuzsanna Jakab. 2018. 'Primary health care for the 21st century, universal health coverage, and the sustainable development goals.' *The Lancet* 392 (10156):1371–1372.

Gibbs, Paul. 2015. 'Transdisciplinarity as epistemology, ontology or principles of practical judgement.' In *Transdisciplinary professional learning and practice*, edited by P. Gibbs, 151–164. Cham: Springer.

Greenhalgh, T. 2008. 'Thirty years on from Alma-Ata: Where have we come from? Where are we going?' *The British Journal of General Practice: The Journal of the Royal College of General Practitioners* 58:798–804. doi:10.3399/bjgp08X342679.

Gunn, J.M., V.J. Palmer, L. Naccarella, R. Kokanovic, C.J. Pope, J. Lathlean, and K. Stange. 2008. 'The promise and pitfalls of generalism in achieving the Alma-Ata vision of health for all.' *Medical Journal of Australia* 189 (2):110–112.

Haslam, Nick. 2016. 'Concept creep: Psychology's expanding concepts of harm and pathology.' *Psychological Inquiry* 27 (1):1–17.

Hunter, Puggy (Arnold). 1999. 'Searching for a new way of thinking in Aboriginal health.' *NACCHO News* 3 (July):1–2.

Hunter, Puggy (Arnold). 2001. *Collected quotes* (unpublished). edited by Kimberly Aboriginal Medical Services Council. Kimberly.

Kirkengen, Anna Luise. 2005. 'Encountering particulars: A life in medicine.' *The Permanente Journal* 9 (3):19.

Kirkengen, Anna Luise, and Eline Thornquist. 2012. 'The lived body as a medical topic: An argument for an ethically informed epistemology.' *Journal of Evaluation in Clinical Practice* 18 (5):1095–1101.

Kluft, Richard P. 2015. *X marks the spot: Psychoform and Somatoform dissociative symptoms open the door to the treatment of dissociative disorders.'* ISSTD Day workshop, Sydney, Australia.

Maslow, A.H. 1954. *Motivation and personality third edition.* Edited by R. Frager, J. Fadiman, C. McReynolds, and R. Cox. New York: Harper Collins Publishers.

McDade, Thomas W. 2008. 'Challenges and opportunities for integrative health research in the context of culture: A commentary on Gersten.' *Social Science & Medicine* 66 (3):520–524.

McWhinney, Ian, M. Stewart, J.B. Brown, W.W. Weston, C.L. McWilliam, and T.R. Freeman. 1995. *Patient-centered medicine. Transforming the clinical method.* Thousand Oaks, CA: Sage.

Nouwen, Henri J.M. 1979. *The wounded healer: Ministry in contemporary society.* New York: Doubleday.

Polk, Merritt. 2014. 'Achieving the promise of transdisciplinarity: A critical exploration of the relationship between transdisciplinary research and societal problem solving.' *Sustainability Science* 9 (4):439–451.

Rappoport, Alan. 1997. 'The patient's search for safety: The organizing principle in psychotherapy.' *Psychotherapy: Theory, Research, Practice, Training* 34 (3):250–261.

Schön, Donald A. 1995. *The reflective practitioner: How professionals think in action.* Vol. 5126. London: Basic books.

Tinetti, Mary E., and Terri Fried. 2004. 'The end of the disease era.' *The American Journal of Medicine* 116 (3):179–185.

WHO. 1978. *The declaration of Alma Ata.* International Conference on Primary Health Care, Alma Ata, USSR, 6–12 September.

Appendices

Appendix I: *Sense of safety dynamics*: Reflection questions for the practitioner

These tables are presented as a prompt for practitioners who want to learn how to attend to the *sense of safety dynamics* in their consultations. They are framed as questions that you can ask yourself or adapt to use in your particular setting. These questions are prompts for reflective practice.

Table AI.i Broad Awareness

BROAD AWARENESS
A form of attention that includes active concurrent intuitive awareness of multiple aspects of self, other and context
Stakeholders words that describe *broad awareness*
'Feeling secure within myself, my community and the wider world' (mhc)   'Feeling safe – for my culture, spirit, identity' (ia)   'Feeling (emotionally and bodily) safe in this particular place, this particular time, with this particular person' (gp)   'Feeling in control of own life, feeling of having supportive people around you, not feeling threatened – now or as a feeling that comes with you from your past' (mhc)   'Not feeling any threat regarding your body, mind and spirit; feeling safe in all aspects of life, being respected for your mind, body, spirit' (le)
Potential questions to raise awareness of the skill of *broad awareness*:
Are you able to enjoy beauty and sorrow in your environment?   Are you open and curious to learn about other people's cultures and experiences?   Can you stay aware that other people have parts of them that they do not speak or want to present to you?   Can you tune in to others through dialogue?   Can you stay aware of yourself when you are near others?   Do you notice when you are hungry, thirsty, tired or tense?   Can you be aware of both your body's internal and external sensations?   Do you ever feel smaller, younger or more vulnerable than you are?   Do you get triggered into flashbacks or confusion with unwanted blank moments of consciousness?   Can you feel and describe your emotions?   Can you attend to both the positive strengths and capacity and negative imperfections, pain or regret inside you?   Can you notice and allow the dialectic of opposing or ambivalent desires or opinions inside you?   Can you attend to the dialogue of your own inner voices?   Can you adapt and accept the questions, doubts and uncertainties in your spirit or meaning-making, as well as the knowing, faith and trust?   Is there a coherent flow to the stories you know about your life?

(Continued)

Table AI.i (Continued) *Broad Awareness*

Reminders for practitioners about *broad awareness*

Practice holding an open, curious attitude to both objective and subjective information

Notice yourself and your body as well as the person you are caring for

Tune in to your own needs, feelings, values and priorities

Notice when the consultation drifts towards a narrow focus – what are you missing or not attending to?

Has the patient's tone of voice or body posture changed to be more focussed on something?

Are they telling a story without accompanying expected emotional or physical responses? Are they numb or bored or disinterested or overly positive?

Keep an awareness of the person's strengths and agency as well as suffering

Keep an awareness of the past, present and future

Keep an awareness of the view of the therapeutic relationship from your and the other person's point of view

Learn to sense transference and countertransference

Beware of narrow focus

Remember to attend to the whole person – across each of the seven domains (environment, social climate, relationships, body, inner experiences, sense of self, meaning and spirit.

Table AI.ii Calm Sense-Making

CALM SENSE-MAKING

Clear-headed, intuitive making sense of self, relationships and environment as part of a wider story

Stakeholders words that describe *calm sense-making*

Being aware and clear-headed

'Bodily sense of calmness – being able to think clearly and creatively' (mhc)

'Being present' (ia)

'Still themselves and allow whatever thoughts that were rubbing around to flow through them' (ia)

'Able to relax and thereby think more clearly'(mhc)

Noticing broadly

'Reflective' (gp)

'Remember my past' (le)

'Perception' (mhc)

'I know how to recognise that I feel threatened' (gp)

Knowing intuitively

'I'll go down into this, I will start to compute inside myself and I'm not even aware of it' (ia)

'What's behind your body language?' (le)

'Can smell, hear, sense … the body holds everything' (ia)

Organising and making sense

'We live storied lives … we organise our experiences into stories as we share our life interactively' (ia)

'Need to learn to contain' (gp)

'Filter it through the maps in their mind' (gp)

'Feeling held and whole' (gp)

(Continued)

Table Al .i i (Continued) *Calm Sense-Making*

Potential questions to raise awareness of the skill of *calm sense-making*

I find time outside, the seasons and rhythms of the day are soothing
I feel I have a place in my community
I participate in rituals, traditions and creativity that help me make sense of my world
Storytelling, play and music help me understand my life and the world around me
I can reminisce about my life without feeling like I am reliving it
My history is connected – there are no confusing gaps in the story
I can feel safe near to someone else
I can sense other's feelings through their tone of voice, facial expressions or body movements
I can talk problems through with people in my life
I don't have confusing or secretive relationships
I feel pretty connected to my body, senses and emotions
I can calm my body down with breathing, tapping, dancing or other forms of exercise
I usually assess situations pretty accurately – my gut feelings are reliable
I am pretty good at understanding myself and other people
I don't feel disconnection or fragmented on the inside
I am good at following through on my own decisions
I know I who I am – I experience myself as the same person in different settings
I have ways to make sense of the transcendent world through philosophy, meditation, prayer or worship

Reminders for practitioners about *calm sense-making*

How coherent is this person's account of their story?
Do their sentences flow and feel ordered?
Do they speak in different tones and intensity of voice with patterned different facial expressions at times?
Do they relate stories where their actions have not matched their intentions?
Do they dress very differently or rigidly the same?
Are they able to organise their time, money and personal hygiene?
Are they settled in a network of relationships?
Do they seem to be able to understand and connect to other people?
Do they seem connected to the wider world in an authentic engaged way?
Can they see the patterns of behaviour that have affected their family?
Have they acknowledged their grief or disappointments?
Do they seem to have mixed feelings towards people close to them?
How are they handling regrets in their life?
Can they include both positive and negative emotions in their descriptions?
Do they express a sense of peace or feeling their life makes sense?
Do they have a sense of hope or purpose?
Do they have a sense of humour or are they focussed and rigid?
Do you feel confused when you are with them?
Has this consultation made you feel fragmented or distracted you from something?
Are you feeling agitated as a result of this meeting?
Can you get a sense of who they are or do you feel like they are 'missing' in some way?

Table AI.iii Respectful Connection

RESPECTFUL CONNECTION

Attuned trusting connecting relationships with self, others, wider community and country

Stakeholders words that describe *respectful connection*

Available and trustworthy

'Honest, congruent, empathetic, genuine' (mhc)
'Presence, attachment – not too close or too far from the other' (mhc)
'Respectful interaction' (gp)
'Cannot underestimate connection to country' (ia)

Tuned in to

'Somebody that gets you and that you can test out your perceptions with' (mhc)
'Truly hearing the person's story' (ia)
'Attunement, attachment, vibration, parents behaviour' (ia)
'Spend-time' (le)

With you/on your side

'Able to allow others to safely be who they are and address misunderstandings respectfully' (gp)
'Intimacy and equality of the relationships' (mhc)
'Belonging, trust' (mhc)
'Walk journey together' (gp)
'If I'm on my own – will I trust myself' (gp)

Potential questions to raise awareness of the skill of *respectful connection*

Do you feel a connection to country or to nature?
Do people connect to you in disrespectful ways – like racism, or injustice?
Is there inequity in how resources, housing, water, food and sanitation are shared in your part of the world?
Are other people disrespected in your community or workplace?
Do feel your culture is respected by your community?
Do you participate in customs that communicate respect to elders and other people you meet?
Is it normal for people's opinions and wishes to be ignored or ghosted in your home or online?
Are the advertising images around you respectful of other people's dignity?
Is the online world you are part of respectful of other people, their images and words?
Do have to witness other people being bullied in your online or analogue worlds?
Do you experience or participate in secrecy, dishonesty, slander or betrayal of others?
Do you experience or participate in taking advantage of others or seeing them as objects to be watched, used, touched, invaded, disconnected from or exploited?
Do you honour others with being available, listening, tuning in and being present?
Do you intentionally include people who are different or lonely?
Can you feel empathy or love towards other people?
Are you careful not to take or do anything without the other person's consent?
Are there respectful reciprocal relationships and conversations around you?
Do you experience coercion, feeling trapped or manipulated in your close relationships?
Do you feel people withdraw from you and you feel alone?
Do people connect to you emotionally so you feel affection and trust?
Do you offer nurture and kindness towards your body?
Do you notice what your body needs, including rest?
Do you respect your interaction with your world through creating or making things?
Can you connect respectful with your own longings or desires?
Do you make decisions without internal recriminations or ignoring?
Do you shame yourself or can you sense inner compassion and kindness?
Do you ignored or minimise your dreams or opinions or gut feelings?
Do you have voices or thoughts that you routinely ignore or attack?
Do you act according to your own values – or do you betray them?
Can you connect to something deeply valuable to you through worship or prayer?
Do you believe in yourself?

(Continued)

Table AI .ii i (Continued) *Respectful Connection*

Reminders for practitioners about *respectful connection*

Do they find beauty or refreshment in nature?
Are the relationships around them online and face-to-face respectful and encouraging?
Is there evidence that they care for their body?
Is there evidence that they ignore their own needs?
Are you noticing your own needs?
Is there any evidence of emotional neglect or abuse in this person's life?
Is there evidence of parental sensitivity and responsiveness to this person?
Do they say words against themselves (like 'stupid', 'idiot', 'bossy-boots', 'lazy') that imply an internal lack of respect?
Do you sense self-loathing or self-hatred in their inner dialogue?
Are you able to maintain respect towards this person even though they are defensive, aggressive or rude?
Can you maintain respect toward this person even when you disagree?
Are you able to honour your own experience and expertise in this moment?
Is all of you OK with this decision
Does this decision sit well with your values and intuition?

Table AI.iv Capable Engagement

CAPABLE ENGAGEMENT

Dynamic interplay of self, other and context that encourages movement towards confident self-expression, engagement and purpose – being Safe Enough to Grow

Stakeholders words that describe *capable engagement*

Freedom to move, grow and learn
'Free to engage' (mhc)
'Given the opportunity to learn and 'fail' and be encouraged to keep learning' (mhc)
'Even if they're not in a relationship where they've been restricted, do they restrict themselves?' (gp)
Having a say
'You feel safe enough to just state your perceptions about things' (mhc)
'Having a voice' (mhc)
'Ability to negotiate sexual relationship' (gp)
'Body language' (mhc)
'Behaviour is language … symptom is story' (ia)
'Express self openly/honestly' (le)
Positive direction
'Meaningful work or creativity' (gp)
'Agency' (gp)
'The sense of values and living towards your values' (mhc)
'Sense of purpose' (gp)
'Automatically dance, sing, that stuff, loss and trauma rituals and practices of indigenous people' (ia)

(Continued)

Table AI.iv (Continued) *Capable Engagement*

Potential questions to raise awareness of the skill of *capable engagement*

I feel I can influence and contribute to my home, work, culture and environment
My finances and housing arrangements make me feel safe enough to take on this world
I can engage and influence my community and receive feedback that enables me to contribute
My voice and who I am are welcomed in my family and workplace
I can question, influence, engage with others and still be treated with value and dignity
I can only cope with life with the help of substances
I feel encouraged and trusting enough to express myself in my close relationships
I feel able to reach out and ask for help from others
I can say no to key people in my life if I need to
I feel strong and connected to my body – my body feels capable
Even when I feel frail, I can move, dance or express myself
I have a sense that I am able to cope in this world
I do not constantly critique myself for not being perfect
I trust my own decision-making
I feel a failure and want to withdraw from life
I am free to be me – to be creative, to feel valid, valued and able
I belong in an existential way that means I can create, question and initiate change in my world
I can't cope with life and make it work for me
I feel endorsed to give my unique contribution to the world

Reminders for practitioners about *capable engagement*

Do processes for getting an appointment offer choice and agency?
Do you sense that other people feel free to be creative and offer new initiatives?
Do you see evidence that other people are able to disagree with you?
Do you encourage each person's active involvement in their life?
Do you make decisions collaboratively?
Do you sense that the other person is growing?
Do you expect appropriate risk-taking or encourage avoidance of risk?

Table AI.v Owning Yourself

OWNING YOURSELF

Dynamic of feeling comfortable, capable and 'with' (aligned to) your whole self

Stakeholders words that describe *owning yourself*

With yourself
'With ourselves' (le)
'Capacity to self-reflect' (mhc)
'A fuller picture of you' (le)
Capacity acknowledged
'Agency to address a threat … agency to make your world safer' (gp)
'Confidence in ability to cope' (mhc)
Feeling comfortable
'Able to relax, reduce monitoring my environment' (mhc)
'Sense bodily calm' (mhc)
'OK to make mistakes' (gp)

(Continued)

Table AI.v (Continued) *Owning Yourself*

Potential questions to raise awareness of the skill of *owning yourself*

I am aware of my impact on my environment
My opinions and ideas are valued in my community
I value and do not feel dominated by my culture
I feel intimidated and excluded in my own community or workplace
I lose a sense of myself when I am near someone else
I find it hard to be calm when other people are disappointed
I find it hard to resist peer pressure
I am ok with being myself – different to those around me
I take care of my body with exercise, nutrition, hygiene and sleep
I am comfortable living in my body
I feel capable of taking responsibility for myself
I take time to understand my own intuitions, sensations and emotions
Can experience safe moments of 'flow' as enjoyable
Bad things always happen to me
I feel a sense of belonging towards myself
I know and live by my own values, dreams and hopes

Reminders for practitioners about *owning yourself*

Do you have a sense that this person is not in tune with themselves?
Do you sense they do not feel capable to act in line with their values?
When they described experiences or emotions do they seem able to reflect and understand themselves in perspective?
Do they seem able to stand on their own two feet even when others disagree?
Do they carry shame or inner disconnection?
Do you sense that they are disowning themselves?
Do you sense that there are other constraints on them expressing themselves?
Do you have a sense that you are feeling internally unified over any decisions made here?
Are you feeling comfortable in yourself?
Are you caring for your own body and soul?

Reference

Northoff, G., F. Bermpohl, F. Schoeneich, and H. Boeker. 2007. 'How does our brain constitute defense mechanisms? First-person neuroscience and psychoanalysis.' *Psychotherapy and Psychosomatics* 76 (3): 141–53.

Appendix II: Resource for frontline staff during COVID-19

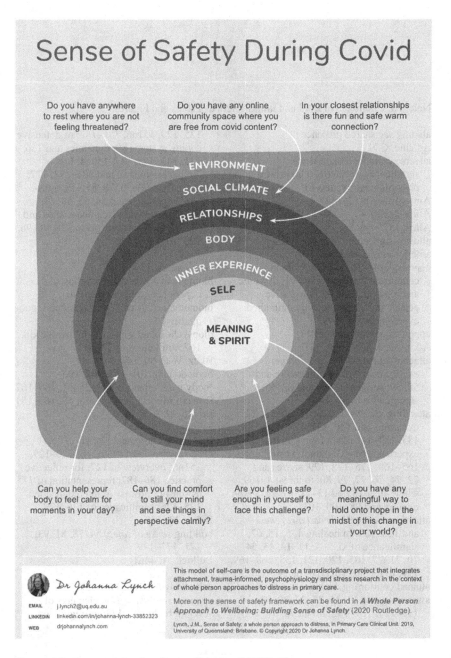

Figure AII.i Resource for frontline staff during COVID-19.

Index

Printed in the United States
By Bookmasters